VIROLOGY MONOGRAPHS

DIE VIRUSFORSCHUNG IN EINZELDARSTELLUNGEN

CONTINUING / FORTFÜHRUNG VON
HANDBOOK OF VIRUS RESEARCH
HANDBUCH DER VIRUSFORSCHUNG
FOUNDED BY / BEGRÜNDET VON
R. DOERR

EDITED BY / HERAUSGEGEBEN VON

S. GARD · C. HALLAUER · K. F. MEYER

12

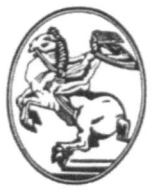

1972

SPRINGER-VERLAG WIEN GMBH

VARICELLA VIRUS

BY

D. TAYLOR-ROBINSON AND ANNE E. CAUNT

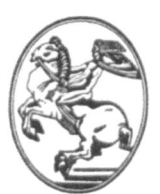

1972

SPRINGER-VERLAG WIEN GMBH

© 1972 by Springer-Verlag Wien
Ursprünglich erschienen bei Springer-Verlag Wien New York 1972
Softcover reprint of the hardcover 1st edition 1972

Library of Congress Catalog Card Number 72-79604
Printer: R. Spies & Co., A-1050 Wien

ISBN 978-3-7091-3429-0   ISBN 978-3-7091-3427-6 (eBook)
DOI 10.1007/978-3-7091-3427-6

Varicella Virus

By

D. Taylor - Robinson

M. R. C. Clinical Research Centre,
Division of Communicable Diseases, Harrow, Middlesex, England

and

Anne E. Caunt

Department of Medical Microbiology,
New Medical School, University of Liverpool, England

With 10 Figures

Table of Contents

I. Introduction and Nomenclature

Varicella virus causes two distinct clinical conditions, chickenpox and herpes zoster. Chickenpox, as varicella is commonly known, is a highly infectious disease which, when introduced by either chickenpox or herpes zoster cases, spreads rapidly in a susceptible population. On the other hand, epidemiological studies have failed to show that herpes zoster is acquired by contact with other cases of herpes zoster or cases of chickenpox. The sporadic occurrence of zoster has led to the hypothesis that this disease represents a reactivation of a latent infection following chickenpox.

The viruses isolated from the two conditions appear from laboratory and epidemiological studies to be identical and this led WELLER (1958) to use the name varicella-zoster virus, a term which has been adopted by many subsequent investigators. However, if zoster results from reactivation of a latent infection with varicella virus it seems reasonable to call the causative agent of both clinical conditions varicella virus and this we shall do in this review. This is in accordance with the nomenclature suggested by ANDREWES (1964) who called the virus *Herpesvirus varicellae*. It also follows the nomenclature of *Herpesvirus hominis (simplex)* which is called by that name regardless of whether it is isolated from primary or recurrent infections.

The name "chickenpox" is derived from the French "chiche" (chick-pea), denoting a small pock, less than a pea in size. Since the causative agent is a member of the herpesvirus group it is unfortunate that the disease is called chickenpox which erroneously suggests a relationship with the poxvirus group. "Varicella" is an irregular diminutive of variola (smallpox) from the Latin *"varius"*, various or mottled. We have found it convenient to use the name chickenpox for the clinical disease and to reserve the term varicella for the causative agent.

The name "zoster" or "zona" comes from the Greek ζωστήρ (a girdle) and refers to the fact that the skin lesions on the trunk spread around it like a girdle. "Herpes", from the Greek ἕρπειν (to creep) is a generic term which has been applied to acute vesiculating inflammatory lesions of the skin, irrespective of aetiology, and as such is misleading. For this reason we have used the term "zoster" alone in referring to the clinical condition in this review. The common name for zoster is shingles, which probably comes from the Latin *"cingere"* to gird (CHRISTIE, 1969).

The association between chickenpox and zoster has intrigued many workers, particularly clinicians, since before the turn of the century and a mass of literature on this clinical relationship has accumulated. In this review clinical data are included where they are pertinent to an understanding of the pathogenesis of the diseases and in such instances the literature is cited in some detail. In other clinical areas, such as disease complications, the literature is not cited in full but reference is made to other reviews of the subject.

Laboratory studies have not so far produced any direct evidence for virus latency following chickenpox. However, the immunological response, even in first attacks of zoster, is of the type which follows a second antigenic stimulus. Such laboratory studies, and those concerning varicella virus itself, are the major concern of this review and in this field an attempt has been made to obtain as complete a bibliography as possible up to 1971. We have also drawn upon the reviews of VAN ROOYEN and RHODES (1948), DOWNIE (1959), GORDON (1962), WENNER and LOU (1963), WELLER (1965), EICHENWALD et al. (1967), PLUMMER (1967), and MORTON (1968).

II. History

Zoster was described in very early medical literature whereas chickenpox was confused with smallpox, the clinical differentiation apparently being made by HEBERDEN in 1767 (GORDON, 1962; WELLER, 1965). VON BÓKAY, who in 1892 reported the occurrence of chickenpox following cases of zoster in two families (v. BÓKAY, 1909), was the first to draw attention to this association. Since then this observation has been made repeatedly and there is now no doubt that zoster is another clinical manifestation of infection by the virus (varicella) which causes chickenpox.

Laboratory studies of the virus have been hampered by the insusceptibility of small common laboratory animals. RIVERS (1926) inoculated chickenpox vesicle fluid into the testicles of immature vervet monkeys and observed intranuclear inclusions in the local lesions so produced. This effect appeared to be a specific response to the virus as it did not occur when the inoculum was first mixed with serum from persons who were convalescent from chickenpox (RIVERS, 1927). No other animals, except man, have been shown to be infected with varicella virus.

Varicella virus does not grow in chick tissues in fertile eggs but evidence of propagation of the virus from zoster vesicle fluid in human skin grafted on the chorio-allantois of hens' eggs was reported by GOODPASTURE and ANDERSON (1944) and BLANK et al. (1948). However, laboratory studies on a large scale only became possible when virus was isolated in suspended tissue cultures by WELLER and STODDARD (1952) from vesicle fluids taken from cases of chickenpox or zoster. Subsequently, the isolation of varicella virus from vesicle fluid and its propagation in monolayer cultures of various human and simian tissues was described (WELLER, 1953; WELLER et al., 1958; TAYLOR-ROBINSON, 1959) but under these conditions the virus remained strictly cell-associated, and cell-free, infectious virus could not be obtained. Virus grown in this way was, therefore, not suitable for direct study of its chemical or physical properties and, although it was used in neutralization tests (WELLER and WITTON, 1958), these were neither quantitative or easy to perform. The finding that cell-free virus could be obtained under suitable conditions from primary cultures of infected human thyroid cells (CAUNT, 1963; CAUNT and TAYLOR-ROBINSON, 1964) has made possible more extensive studies of the virus (SHAW, 1968), the performance of quantitative neutralization tests (CAUNT and SHAW, 1969) and the investigation of possible antigenic relationships between varicella and herpes simplex viruses (SCHMIDT et al., 1969).

In the absence of methods for growing varicella virus, the first serological studies were performed using crusts or vesicle fluids as antigens. NETTER and URBAIN (1926) and BRAIN (1933) did complement-fixation tests using such antigens from chickenpox and zoster cases and found that they reacted equally well with convalescent, but not acute, sera from either disease. The subsequent growth of virus in tissue culture provided an alternative source of antigen, even in the absence of cell-free virus, and it was shown to be as potent and as specific as vesicle fluid antigens in complement-fixation and gel-diffusion tests (WELLER and WITTON, 1958; TAYLOR-ROBINSON and DOWNIE, 1959; TAYLOR-ROBINSON and RONDLE, 1959). The fluorescent-antibody technique was particularly useful in establishing the identity of virus isolates which remained cell-associated (WELLER and COONS, 1954). Thus a variety of laboratory methods is now available for the study of varicella virus infection in man, and although these have not yet been widely applied it seems likely that they will eventually help to elucidate the pathogenesis and epidemiology of chickenpox and zoster infections which at present must be deduced mainly from clinical observations.

III. Classification

The herpesvirus group as defined by ANDREWES (1964) consists of viruses with the following characteristics:
1. icosahedral with 162 capsomeres and usually enveloped
2. size: 100—150 mµ
3. contain DNA
4. ether sensitive
5. haemagglutinin not demonstrable
6. no antigen common to the whole group but some antigenic cross-reactions
7. all grow in tissue culture and some in eggs also
8. synthesis begins in the nucleus of the host cell
9. produce proliferative lesions which soon become necrotic.
10. characteristic intranuclear inclusions of Cowdry's type A found.
11. many members grow in the central nervous system (CNS) and some travel along nerves to reach the CNS.

Varicella virus meets these criteria and was included in the group as *Herpesvirus varicellae* by ANDREWES (1964) and by ANDREWES and PEREIRA (1967). PLUMMER (1967) also included varicella virus in the herpesvirus group on the grounds of its morphology, envelopment, DNA content and replication in the nucleus of the host cell. Varicella virus is also included in the herpesvirus group by CRANDELL (1967) who used ANDREWES' (1964) criteria to define the group. MELNICK *et al.* (1964) suggested that the herpesviruses might be divided into two groups, A and B. Viruses in Group A, typified by *Herpesvirus hominis (simplex)* are liberated from cells in infectious form while those in Group B, including varicella virus and cytomegalovirus, remain cell-associated in tissue cultures. The feasibility of such a division has been questioned by PLUMMER (1967) since there is no clear cut distinction between the two groups but rather a spectrum of ability to produce free virus in tissue culture. The term "group B herpesvirus" may also be confused with herpes B virus *(Herpesvirus simiae)* and hence we have not used it in this review.

IV. Properties of the Virion

A. Morphology

1. Virus in Vesicle Fluid

Minute particles in chickenpox vesicle fluid were first seen by ARAGÃO (1911) using light microscopy. PASCHEN (1917, 1919) recognized that these were probably virus particles and later similar particles were demonstrated in zoster vesicle fluid (PASCHEN, 1933; TANIGUCHI et al., 1934). AMIES (1933, 1934) described staining methods which showed that virus particles in zoster and chickenpox vesicle fluids were morphologically alike. VAN ROOYEN and ILLINGWORTH (1944) found it possible to distinguish chickenpox from smallpox by examining stained smears from vesicles. They described varicella elementary bodies as 0.125—0.175 µ in diameter, these being smaller and much less numerous in the smears than were virus particles from smallpox vesicles.

RUSKA (1943 a, b), in the first electron microscope study of chickenpox vesicle fluid, described the virus particles as round or polygonal with a central dot and distinguished them from the brick-shaped particles of the poxviruses. NAGLER and RAKE (1948), however, using a metal shadowing technique described varicella virus particles as brick-shaped and distinguished them from those of poxviruses only by their smaller size (average size of varicella virus was 210×238 mµ and of variola virus was 244×302 mµ). RAKE et al. (1948) examined chickenpox and zoster vesicle fluids by the same techniques and found similar brick-shaped particles in each. The same metal shadowing technique was used by FARRANT and O'CONNOR (1949) to examine viruses from chickenpox and zoster vesicle fluids and they concluded that the particles which they demonstrated probably represented collapsed spheres or ellipsoids. EVANS and MELNICK (1949) also described spherical

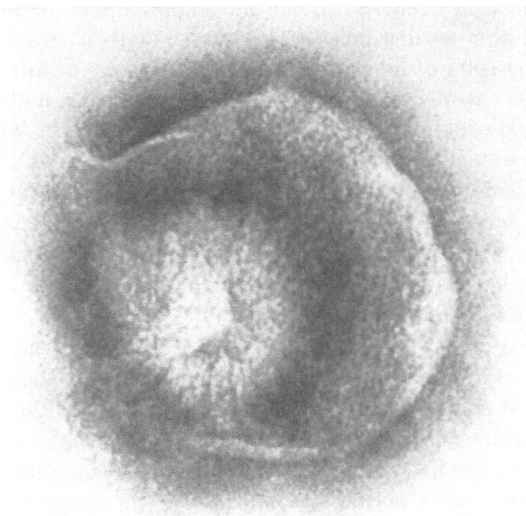

Fig. 1. Varicella virus particle from chickenpox vesicle fluid. Negative staining with phosphotungstic acid. $\times 302{,}500$

particles from chickenpox and zoster vesicle fluids and from zoster cerebrospinal fluid and pointed out their similarity to herpes simplex virus from vesicle fluid. REAGAN et al. (1953) demonstrated spherical virus particles (diameter 175 mμ) in sera of monkeys thought to be infected with varicella virus, but since generalized infection of monkeys has never been confirmed it seems likely that this could have been a latent simian herpesvirus rather than varicella.

ALMEIDA et al. (1962) used negative staining with phosphotungstic acid to make detailed observations of varicella virus from vesicle fluid (Fig. 1). The virion consists of a central body surrounded by a capsid composed of hollow capsomeres which in turn is surrounded by a granular zone, and enveloped by a membrane with filamentous projections about 8 mμ long on its outer surface. The diameter of the capsid is about 95 mμ but the total diameter of the enveloped particle is 200 mμ. The capsid resembles that of herpes simplex virus in having the symmetry characteristics of an icosahedron with a 5:3:2 axial symmetry. There are 5 capsomeres along one edge and the total number of capsomeres has therefore been deduced to be 162. Similar particles have been found in zoster vesicle fluid (WILLIAMS et al., 1962; HERZBERG et al., 1963 b). The latter authors suggested that this negative-staining technique enabled poxviruses to be distinguished from varicella virus and CRUICKSHANK et al. (1966) used it diagnostically to distinguish varicella virus from smallpox virus in specimens of vesicle fluids or crusts.

Particles, similar in appearance to those described by ALMEIDA et al. (1962), were observed in cell-free varicella virus preparations obtained from infected human thyroid tissue cultures (SHAW, 1968).

2. Virus in Tissue Cells

The appearance in the electron microscope of varicella virus in thin sections of early skin lesions and in tissue cultures of human embryo fibroblast cells was described by TOURNIER et al. (1957). They found that in both materials the earliest signs of virus infection occurred in the nucleus of infected cells, first as areas of granularity and later as distinct particles each with a single membrane. These particles were 70—100 mμ in diameter. At a later stage of infection particles were also found in the cytoplasm, but in this situation they had acquired a second membrane thus enlarging their diameter to 100—160 mμ. These particles were also found on the external surfaces of cells in tissue culture, although no infectious virus could be demonstrated in the culture fluids. The extracellular particles always had two membranes and an average diameter of 150—200 mμ. These authors also drew attention to the similarity of varicella virus to herpes simplex (HS) virus and to herpes B virus both in morphology and also in its replication in the nucleus of the infected cell.

The appearance of virus in skin lesions of zoster was described by DOHI et al. (1961) as an oval particle often with a small nucleoid and surrounded by one or two membranes. Particles within the nucleus were smaller than those in the cytoplasm. LUTZNER (1962, 1963), however, described spherical virus particles in a biopsy of a skin lesion of zoster. He found particles with double membranes in the nuclei of infected cells as well as in the cytoplasm and in the extra-cellular spaces. MONTALDO et al. (1966) described the presence of uniform virus particles with a diameter of 150—160 mμ in chickenpox biopsy material, mainly within the giant cells

Table 1. *Estimations of Size of Varicella Virus*

Reference	Material examined	Total virus diameter (mμ)	Diameter of naked virion (mμ)	Diameter of inner core (mμ)
RUSKA, 1943	CP and Z vesicle fluid	150	—	"central thickening" 50
NAGLER and RAKE, 1948	CP vesicle fluid	210 × 238	—	—
FARRANT and O'CONNOR, 1949	CP vesicle fluid	175—245[1]		
	Z vesicle fluid	253		
EVANS and MELNICK, 1949	CP vesicle fluid	245 (range 160—320)		
	Z vesicle fluid	230		
	Z cerebrospinal fluid	224		
ALMEIDA et al., 1962	CP vesicle fluid	200	95	
WILLIAMS et al., 1962	Z vesicle fluid	200	95	
HERZBERG et al., 1963	Z vesicle fluid	200	90—100	
SHAW, 1968	CP, Z in thyroid TC	200	100	
DOHI et al., 1961	Z skin section	80—90 × 140—180	60—90 × 80—100	20
LUTZNER, 1962	Z skin biopsy	160		50
MONTALDO et al., 1966	CP skin biopsy	150—160		
KIMURA et al., 1972	CP skin biopsy	180—200	100[2]	
ESIRI and TOMLINSON, 1972	Z skin and nerve section	116—140	70—80[2]	34—42
TOURNIER et al., 1957	CP in human fibroblast TC	150—200		
BECKER et al., 1965	Z in human embryo lung fibroblast TC	150 (average)	90	45
ACHONG and MEURISSE, 1968	CP in human amnion TC	120	90[2]	45
COOK and STEVENS, 1968	CP in human amnion TC	115[3]	81—90[3]	
TAWARA and OGIWARA, 1969	CP in VERO (vervet monkey embryo) TC	190—220	90—110	70—90

CP = chickenpox; Z = zoster; TC = tissue culture.

[1] Depended on method of fixation used. [2] Single envelope. [3] Estimated from photographs.

in chickenpox vesicles. KIMURA et al. (1972) studied chickenpox skin biopsies. In the nuclei of cells, the particles had a single membrane, were 100 mμ in diameter, and were sometimes hexagonal. In association with these, tubular structures were seen which were about 30 mμ in width; these were possibly aberrant virus forms. Budding of particles from the inner nuclear membrane and from the membrane of cytoplasmic vacuoles seemed to occur. Single membrane particles were seen occasionally in the cytoplasm but here the particles mostly had double membranes and were 180 to 200 mμ in diameter. ESIRI and TOMLINSON (1971) detected virus particles in autopsy material from a case of ophthalmic zoster. Particles were present in the nuclei and cytoplasm of epidermal cells, the cytoplasm of perineurial cells and the nuclei and cytoplasm of Schwann cells of the frontal nerve, and likewise in the ganglion and satellite cells of the trigeminal ganglion. Particles with a single outer membrane, found almost exclusively in the nuclei, had an average diameter of 80 mμ in epidermal cells, 70 mμ in Schwann cells and 78 mμ in ganglion cells. Double membraned particles in the cytoplasm or outside cells had a diameter of 140 mμ in the epidermis and 116 and 136 mμ in Schwann and ganglion cells respectively. The nucleoid diameter was 42 mμ in the skin and 34 mμ in Schwann and ganglion cells.

In addition to the observations of TOURNIER et al. (1957) on the appearance of virus in tissue cultures of human embryo cells mentioned above, virus particles have also been observed in ultra-thin sections of infected tissue cultures by BECKER et al. (1965), ACHONG and MEURISSE (1968), COOK and STEVENS (1968) and TAWARA and OGIWARA (1969). The development of these particles will be described more fully in the section on cytopathic effects (CPE) produced by the virus in tissue culture.

The observations made in studies with the electron microscope are summarized in Table 1. These suggest that the virion has a central core 45—50 mμ in diameter, surrounded by a capsid and this nucleocapsid has a diameter of 95—100 mμ. The enveloped particle is larger than this and diameters of 150—240 mμ are quoted.

B. Chemical and Physical Properties

1. Chemical Composition

The chemical composition of varicella virus has not been studied by conventional biochemical methods of analysis, but RAPP and VANDERSLICE (1964) showed that the spread of virus isolated from a case of zoster was inhibited in tissue culture in the presence of IUDR which is known to inhibit DNA but not RNA viruses. Subsequently, RAPP (1964) showed that the virus was inhibited also by cytosine arabinoside and that the dosage of either this or IUDR required, and the degree of suppression obtained, was the same as for herpes simplex virus, which is known to contain DNA. Inhibition by IUDR of the growth of varicella virus isolated from both chickenpox and zoster cases was demonstrated also by RAWLS et al. (1964).

A more direct demonstration of the nature of the nucleic acid in varicella virions was provided by COOK and STEVENS (1970) who showed that in ultra-thin sections of infected human amnion cells the dense central cores were removed by treatment with DNase but not by RNase.

2. Resistance to Physical and Chemical Agents

a) Thermal Stability

WELLER (1953) recorded that vesicle fluid lost its capacity to infect cells after it had been heated at 60° C for 30 minutes. CAUNT and TAYLOR-ROBINSON (1964) found that virus from vesicle fluid, suspended in 2 per cent calf serum in 199 medium at pH 7.6, showed little if any loss of viability after storage at 37° C for 9 hours and only a 40 per cent loss after 15 hours. Cell-free virus obtained from infected human thyroid cell cultures and stored under the same conditions appeared to be less stable, 50 per cent of the infectious virus being lost after 9 hours at 37° C. SHAW (1968) also used cell-free virus prepared in human thyroid cells and tested its survival at 37° C, room temperature (about 22° C) and 4° C; his results are shown in Table 2.

Table 2. *Lability at Various Temperatures of Varicella Virus Obtained from Infected Human Thyroid Cells*

Time (hours) at indicated temperature	Percentage virus[1] survival at		
	Room temperature (21—24° C)	4° C	36° C
1.5	100	100	100
3	100	75	(21)
5	100	80	32
7	60	80	22
9	57	78	20
12	55	(100)	10
24	20	43	0.1

[1] Virus suspended in PBS containing 2 per cent inactivated calf serum; initial concentration 10^4 pfu/ml.

b) pH Stability

No evidence is available about the effect of pH on cell-free virus particles. GOLD (1965) reported that infected human amnion cells held at room temperature for 60 minutes lost their infectivity if the pH value of the suspending fluid was less than 6.2 or greater than 7.8. HAMPARIAN et al. (1963) also considered varicella virus to be acid labile, that is unstable at pH 3, in tests on infected human embryo fibroblast cells. These results, however, may only reflect the death of the cells used at the more extreme pH values, since in the systems used viable cells are necessary for the transmission of infectious virus.

c) Effect of Ultrasonic Vibration

Since infectious varicella virus can be liberated from some tissue-culture systems by disrupting the cells by ultrasonic vibration, the resistance of the virus to this treatment is of some interest. CAUNT and TAYLOR-ROBINSON (1964) treated cell-free vesicle fluid virus ultrasonically and found that the titre of infectious virus was reduced by 50 per cent in 1 minute and by 75 per cent in 2 minutes but that some virus survived even 10 minutes treatment. When an infected human thyroid cell suspension of 10^6 plaque-forming units (p.f.u.)/ml was treated in this way, the yield of cell-free virus after 2 minutes was usually 10^4 to 10^5. It seems reasonable to suppose that if the cells could be disrupted by a shorter period of treatment then a higher yield of virus might be obtained. SHAW (1968) prepared a virus suspension containing 8×10^4 p.f.u./ml by 30 seconds ultrasonic treatment of infected human thyroid cells. The suspension was centrifuged at low speed to deposit any remaining cells and then subjected to further periods of ultrasonic treatment. There was no fall in the titre of infectious virus after another 30 seconds treatment but after 120 seconds the titre had fallen to 1.6×10^4 p.f.u./ml, a loss approximately equivalent to that found for virus in vesicle fluid by CAUNT and TAYLOR-ROBINSON (1964).

BRUNELL (1967 b) investigated the release of virus from infected human fibroblasts and found that the maximum yield was obtained by ultrasonic treatment for 15 to 30 seconds. Treatment for a longer time caused the virus yield to fall until after 120 seconds it was negligible. This more rapid loss of infectivity than that found by SHAW (1968) probably reflects differences in the apparatus used and in the initial infectious virus titres of the preparations.

d) Sensitivity to Organic Solvents

The infectivity of varicella virus is rapidly destroyed by ether. SHAW (1968) showed that less than 10 p.f.u./ml of varicella virus remained after 4 minutes ether treatment of a suspension which originally contained 3.6×10^4 p.f.u./ml. Similar sensitivity to ether is shown by other herpesviruses.

HERZBERG et al. (1963 a) showed by electron microscope studies of virus from zoster vesicle fluid that the structure of the capsomeres was rapidly destroyed by treatment with methanol. Subsequently, they reported (HERZBERG et al., 1964) that absolute ethanol had a similar effect but that 96 per cent ethanol was less destructive and acetone and petroleum ether were without effect. The infectivity of the virus preparations was not investigated.

e) Trypsin Sensitivity

BRUNELL (1967 b) treated varicella virus, which had been liberated from human embryo lung fibroblasts, with 20 µg/ml of crystalline trypsin for 30 minutes at 25° C and found the titre of infectious virus fell by more than tenfold.

f) Preservation

Cell-free virus in vesicle fluid. WELLER and STODDARD (1952) stored vesicle fluid, usually diluted with sterile fat-free milk, at − 65° C for periods of up to 13 months and still found infectious virus in the fluid. Later, WELLER et al. (1958) reported that they had isolated virus from vesicle fluid stored for as long as $4\,{}^3/_4$ years. TAYLOR-ROBINSON (1959) found that the titre of infectious virus in vesicle fluid fell by less than 50 per cent on storage at −70° C for 75 days.

SÖLTZ-SZÖTS (1964) claimed to have isolated virus from zoster vesicle fluid stored at −20° C for an unspecified time. NETTER (1964), however, recorded the complete loss of infectivity of vesicle fluid after 1 hour at −10° C.

Virus from "organ" cultures. Cell-free virus can be extracted from cultures of fragments of human embryo skin or lung and such virus has been shown to survive storage at −70° C for as long as $6\,{}^1/_2$ years (CAUNT, 1969).

Cell-free virus from tissue-culture cells. CAUNT and TAYLOR-ROBINSON (1964) reported that 10 per cent of infectious varicella virus prepared by ultrasonic disruption of infected human thyroid cells survived storage in 199 medium supplemented with 5 per cent calf serum for 84 days at −70° C, while BRUNELL (1967 b) recorded only a minimal loss of titre of virus prepared from human embryo fibroblasts when it was stored in 10 per cent sorbitol in Hanks' saline for months at −73° C. GÉDER *et al.* (1964—65) found that the titre of infectious virus obtained from human thyroid cells or a continuous line of monkey kidney cells was reduced 25-fold when it was stored in 199 medium for 4 days at −20° C.

Infected tissue-culture cells in which the virus remains cell-associated. WELLER *et al.* (1958) suspended infected tissue-culture cells, from which they were unable to separate free infectious virus, in a mixture of 5 per cent beef embryo extract and 95 per cent bovine amniotic fluid to which 5 per cent horse serum was added. This suspension was frozen rapidly and the cells were still able to infect fresh tissue cultures after storage at −40° to −50° C for 2 months, but subsequently their ability to do so became irregular and unpredictable. The authors suggested that survival of viable cells was necessary for survival of infectious virus and this suggestion received support from the work of ROSANOFF and HEGARTY (1964) who demonstrated that the infectivity of human diploid fibroblast cells survived when they were frozen at −70° C in Eagle's medium which contained 10 per cent calf serum and 5 per cent glycerol, conditions which also preserved the viability of the cells. ROSANOFF (1963) had found previously that glycerol was superior to dimethyl sulphoxide for the preservation of infected cells. RAPP and BENYESH-MELNICK (1963) also recorded that human embryo lung fibroblast cells infected with varicella virus retained their infectivity when suspended in Eagle's medium containing 20 per cent calf serum and 15 per cent glycerol and frozen in liquid nitrogen at −195° C. Later GOLD (1965) showed that viable cells, as defined by their ability to exclude eosin Y, were essential for the initiation of infection by cell suspensions. He recommended rapid freezing of infected human amnion cells in Eagle's medium containing 10 per cent horse serum, and records that such cells were still infectious after storage for 97 days but not 150 days at −20° C and for 255 days at −70° C. MEURISSE (1969) preserved infected human amnion cells by freezing them at −65° C as a monolayer on the glass of the bottle in which they were grown. Bottles were frozen in a position in which the cells were covered with a thin layer of 199 medium containing 10 per cent horse serum. On rapid thawing at 37° C cells capable of transferring infection were recovered up to 3 years later.

C. Antigenic Structure and Serological Techniques

1. Relationship of Virus from Chickenpox to Virus from Zoster

The antigenic structure of varicella virus has been investigated by complement-fixation, agglutination, immunofluorescence, precipitation and neutralization reactions. Early workers used the first two of the tests mentioned and employed vesicle fluids or crusts as their source of antigen and acute and convalescent-phase sera from chickenpox or zoster cases. More recently, complement-fixation, immunofluorescence, precipitation and neutralization tests have been used with antigens or virus produced in tissue culture. Specific immune sera prepared in laboratory animals have been used also. Many of the investigations have aimed at showing the similarity or identity of viruses from cases of chickenpox and zoster and we shall discuss these first and consider the antigenic relationship of varicella to other herpesviruses afterwards.

a) Complement Fixation

DE LANGE (1923) used emulsified crusts from chickenpox vesicles as antigen and showed that this fixed complement in reactions with sera from two cases of chickenpox and from one of zoster. In a series of papers NETTER and URBAIN (NETTER et al., 1924; NETTER and URBAIN, 1924 a, b; NETTER and URBAIN, 1926) showed that complement fixation occurred when crust or vesicle fluid antigens from chickenpox or zoster reacted with convalescent-phase sera from either clinical entity. The tests included sera from 100 zoster and 24 chickenpox patients and the reactions were virtually identical with homologous and heterologous antigens and sera. In addition, reactions between chickenpox or zoster antigens and sera from herpes simplex cases were not detected.

BEDSON and BLAND (1929) demonstrated complement fixation using undiluted serum from 3 convalescent zoster cases and 3 different vesicle fluid antigens. Two of the 3 sera also fixed complement in reactions using CSF, from a supposed case of zoster encephalitis, as antigen. BRAIN (1933) examined sera from 17 chickenpox and 44 zoster cases and confirmed the findings of NETTER and URBAIN concerning the identity of chickenpox and zoster viruses but strongly recommended the use of vesicle fluid as antigen, instead of crust extracts which were frequently anticomplementary. In spite of this, various other workers (LAUDA and SILBERSTERN, 1925; THOMSEN, 1934; HASSKÓ et al., 1938) continued to use crust antigens, since these were more readily available than vesicle fluid; they obtained equivocal results which suggested that either the viruses of chickenpox and zoster were unrelated, or if related not identical. In retrospect it seems likely that in these studies the antigens used were too weak to give reliable results.

WELLER (1953) found that fluids from tissue cultures infected with varicella virus would fix complement in the presence of sera obtained from patients recovering from chickenpox. WELLER and WITTON (1958) described this work in more detail and reported that either tissue-culture fluid concentrated 25 times, or infected human fibroblasts frozen and thawed in veronal buffer, provided satisfactory antigens for complement-fixation tests. Occasionally these antigens were anticomplementary but this could be overcome by heating them at 56° or 60° C for 30 minutes, although this caused some loss of antigenicity. Most of their work was done with tissue-culture fluid antigens, and those prepared with viruses originally isolated from chickenpox or zoster cases gave similar results. Twenty-three chickenpox sera were tested with both chickenpox and zoster antigens; 16 had the same antibody titres, while 5 showed a 2-fold difference and only 2 showed a 4-fold difference between tests using chickenpox and zoster antigens. Among 43 zoster sera, 23 had identical antibody titres, 18 gave a 2-fold difference and again only 2 had 4-fold differences with the two antigens. The specificity of the reaction was also demonstrated. A rise in complement-fixing antibody titre was demonstrated with paired sera from all of 54 cases of chickenpox or zoster but not with paired sera from 4 cases of generalised vaccinia, or 11 of 13 patients with herpes simplex virus infections. In the paired sera of the remaining 2 patients with herpes simplex infections, 2-fold and 4-fold rises in antibody titre were observed.

TAYLOR-ROBINSON and DOWNIE (1959) tested paired sera from chickenpox and zoster patients using both vesicle fluids and tissue-culture fluids as antigens. They found that for any one serum identical results were obtained regardless of whether a chickenpox or zoster antigen was used and they concluded, like WELLER and WITTON, that viruses from the two clinical entities were identical in their complement-fixing antigens. They showed also that if infectious virus was sedimented from vesicle fluid by ultracentrifugation (20,000 r.p.m.; 36,200 × g for 30 minutes), the non-infectious supernatant fluid was still able to fix complement and they presumed that this indicated that the complement-fixing antigen was soluble and unassociated with the virus particle. However, SCHMIDT et al. (1964), in preparing complement-fixing antigen from human embryo diploid skin-muscle cells found that most of it was associated with the cells and that which was present in the culture fluid could be sedimented at 20,000 r.p.m. in 90 minutes. They concluded that there was no soluble antigen separable from the virus particle.

KAPSENBERG (1964) showed no difference in titre when chickenpox and zoster sera were tested in complement-fixation tests against tissue-culture antigens derived from either clinical entity. A similar observation was made by GOLD and GODEK (1965).

b) Agglutination

AMIES (1933) demonstrated that the virus particles in chickenpox vesicle fluids could be agglutinated by sera from convalescent chickenpox patients and PASCHEN (1933) showed the same reaction with virus particles from zoster vesicles and the serum of a convalescent zoster patient. AMIES (1934), in further investigations, tested convalescent-phase chickenpox and zoster sera for agglutinins to viruses in chickenpox and zoster vesicle fluids and found that some, but not all, sera gave cross agglutination.

c) Precipitation

Precipitation lines formed by zoster vesicle fluid and sera from convalescent zoster patients were demonstrated by TAYLOR-ROBINSON and RONDLE (1959) who used the double diffusion technique of OUCHTERLONY (1948). At least 3 distinct lines were observed in this system. An identical pattern was seen with chickenpox vesicle fluid and the same zoster sera and there was a fusion of lines produced by the two systems indicating the identity of the antigen-antibody reactions involved. Tests in which convalescent-phase chickenpox sera and vesicle fluids from either chickenpox or zoster patients were used gave precipitation lines only if the sera were first concentrated 5 times. If fluids from tissue cultures infected with virus derived from either condition were concentrated 25 times, they also precipitated with convalescent zoster and concentrated convalescent chickenpox sera and again the precipitation lines merged in a reaction of identity. It was concluded that viruses isolated from the vesicles of chickenpox and zoster patients had identical antigenic composition.

The results of TRLIFAJOVÁ et al. (1970) who used chickenpox and zoster sera concentrated two-fold and concentrated antigens prepared by freezing and thawing infected tissue-culture cells mainly support this view, but with four of their zoster sera they obtained more lines of precipitation with zoster than with chickenpox antigens.

TAYLOR-ROBINSON and RONDLE (1959) compared the precipitating and complement-fixing abilities of the sera and antigens they used. Their results indicated that precipitating antigens were not the only ones which fixed complement; the two techniques did not necessarily give parallel results. A similar lack of parallelism was noted by CAUNT et al. (1961).

d) Immunofluorescence

The cell-associated nature of varicella virus when it was first grown in tissue culture posed problems in its serological identification. However, WELLER and COONS (1954) showed that convalescent-phase, but not acute-phase, sera from chickenpox and zoster patients reacted with cell cultures infected with viruses from either condition and that these reactions could be demonstrated by using a fluorescein-conjugated rabbit anti-human serum. The same indirect immunofluorescence technique was used by GÉDER et al. (1963) who showed that 6 different isolates of virus from zoster cases reacted equally well with a convalescent- but not an acute-phase serum from one of the cases.

SCHMIDT et al. (1965 b) immunized rhesus monkeys with whole monkey kidney cells infected with varicella virus. They obtained antisera which reacted specifically with tissue-culture cells infected with varicella virus in immunofluorescence tests and with varicella antigens (SCHMIDT et al., 1964) in complement-fixation tests. Specific antisera produced in rabbits by inoculation of virus grown in human fibroblasts and purified by sucrose density gradient centrifugation (KISSLING et al., 1968) also reacted with varicella antigens in complement-fixation tests and with cells infected with varicella virus in immunofluorescence tests. There is no evidence, however, that the same antigens are concerned in these two tests, although SCHMIDT et al. (1965 b) noted that titres of antibody in human serum seemed to decline as rapidly when measured by the indirect immunofluorescence technique as they did when measured by complement fixation.

e) Neutralization Tests

In the initial laboratory studies of varicella virus there was a lack of cell-free infectious virus and hence WELLER and WITTON (1958) attempted neutralization tests using suspensions of varicella virus-infected tissue-culture cells as inocula. They incorporated the test sera at a concentration of 10 per cent in the nutrient medium of the tissue cultures and did not obtain complete neutralization of the cytopathic effects, which is not surprising since the virus was always in the intracellular state. However, in the presence of convalescent-phase sera there was a delay in the time of appearance of foci of infection, the numbers of foci were reduced and their size and subsequent spread were diminished. These workers regularly demonstrated such inhibition of virus effect, whether the virus was derived from chickenpox or zoster cases, by convalescent sera from both diseases and they argued that this was added evidence of the close similarity or identity of the viruses concerned.

TAYLOR-ROBINSON (1959) obtained similar results with infected tissue-culture cells as his source of virus but he also observed complete inhibition of cytopathic effects in tests where vesicle fluid, which contained cell-free virus, was the virus source. In the latter case, convalescent-phase chickenpox and zoster sera completely neutralized the cytopathic effects produced by virus from either clinical entity. It thus appears that virus strains from chickenpox and zoster cases are indistinguishable in these neutralization tests, or indeed by any other serological means. However, it is possible that the methods so far described would not detect minor antigenic differences or strain variation which might be shown, for example, by kinetic neutralization tests. GÉDER et al. (1963) looked for antigenic variation among 6 viruses isolated from different zoster cases. In addition to the indirect immunofluorescence test described in the previous section (p. 16), they also did neutralization tests with the sera (3 paired and 2 acute-phase only) from 5 of the patients from whom the viruses were isolated. They showed slight (4—8 per cent) differences in the neutralizing ability of a patients' serum when it was tested against his own and other virus isolates, but concluded that these differences were not significant and that the 6 viruses isolated were antigenically identical.

2. Relationship of Varicella Virus to Herpes Simplex (HS) Virus

Varicella virus has been included in the herpesvirus group because of its similarity in morphological and other characteristics to members of the group, particularly HS virus (see p. 6). It is, therefore, logical to look for antigenic relationships between varicella virus and other herpesviruses.

There is no evidence from the earlier work for an antigenic relationship between varicella and other viruses. NETTER and URBAIN (1924 b) noted that complement-fixing antigens prepared from extracts of crusts from chickenpox and zoster cases did not fix complement in tests with sera from 9 "normal" subjects including 6 with HS virus infections. BEDSON and BLAND (1929) demonstrated the specificity of their complement-fixation test by showing that antigen prepared from zoster vesicle fluid would not react with serum from a guinea pig hyperimmunized with HS virus and that sera from convalescent zoster patients did not react with HS or vaccinia virus antigens. BRAIN (1933) also noted that neither chickenpox nor zoster convalescent sera fixed complement in tests with HS vesicle fluid.

In their immunofluorescence studies, WELLER and COONS (1954) did not detect a rise in antibody titre to HS virus in tests with paired acute and convalescent chickenpox or zoster sera. The antisera produced by SCHMIDT et al. (1965 b) by immunizing monkeys with varicella virus grown in tissue culture also failed to react in immunofluorescence tests with cells infected with HS virus.

The first hint of the sharing of antigenic components between varicella and HS viruses was the previously mentioned (p. 15) finding of WELLER and WITTON (1958) that paired sera from 2 of their 13 HS cases showed rises in complement-fixing antibody titre when tested with concentrated fluids from varicella virus-infected tissue cultures. This was not the experience of BRUNELL and CASEY (1964) who failed to detect a rise in complement-fixing antibody titre using acute and convalescent HS sera and varicella virus antigens prepared by freezing and thawing infected human embryo fibroblasts. KAPSENBERG (1964) also prepared a varicella complement-fixing antigen from infected human embryo diploid fibroblasts disrupted by ultrasonic vibration, and showed that this antigen did not react with guinea pig anti-HS serum, nor with a human serum which contained antibodies to human cytomegalovirus. It did react, however, with paired sera from 12 of 49 patients with primary HS infections; in these, 4-fold or greater rises in the titre of complement-fixing antibody to varicella virus were demonstrated. This, she suggested, could be due to a sharing of minor antigenic components of the two viruses. Similar results were obtained by SVEDMYR (1965) who used antigen prepared by freezing and thawing varicella virus-infected HeLa cells. This antigen failed to fix complement in tests with guinea pig anti-HS serum but it did in tests with paired acute and convalescent-phase sera from patients with primary HS virus infections; 9 of 14 cases had at least a 4-fold rise in the titre of complement-fixing antibody to varicella virus antigen.

Ross *et al.* (1965 b) examined paired sera from chickenpox and zoster patients for rises in complement-fixing antibody to HS virus and found that 4-fold or greater rises occurred in the sera of 10 of 21 chickenpox and 5 of 19 zoster patients. The rise was usually greater in chickenpox than in zoster illness. Three of the chickenpox and one of the zoster patients had no detectable ($< 1/8$) complement-fixing antibody to HS virus in the acute or convalescent-phase sera. The remaining patients possessed complement-fixing antibody to HS virus but there was no rise in titre during the course of chickenpox or zoster. The sera were also examined for neutralizing antibody to HS virus and a small (< 4-fold) but definite rise in titre was shown in 9 of the chickenpox and 5 of the zoster cases.

The rise in titre of complement-fixing antibody to HS virus occurring in the sera of chickenpox patients was confirmed by SCHAAP and HUISMAN (1968). They found that it occurred in 13 of 25 chickenpox patients where HS virus antibody was present in the acute-phase serum but it did not occur in those devoid of such antibody. A similar heterologous antibody titre rise did not occur in 108 zoster patients whom they studied, except in one from whom both varicella and HS viruses were isolated. It is possible, however, that in these and in the 12 cases of chickenpox for which no antibody titre rise was demonstrated, the acute-phase serum was taken too late (more than 3 days after the onset of the rash) for any further rise to be shown. CAUNT and SHAW (1969) also confirmed the occurrence of a rise in titre of complement-fixing antibody to HS virus in chickenpox patients with pre-existing antibody, but not in chickenpox patients who were not already herpetics or in 2 zoster patients with pre-existing antibody to HS virus. They also failed to show any rise in titre of neutralizing antibody to HS virus even in those chickenpox patients who had pronounced increases in the titre of complement-fixing antibody to HS virus.

A comprehensive investigation into the relationship between varicella and HS viruses was made by SCHMIDT *et al.* (1969) who used complement-fixation, immuno-fluorescence and neutralization tests. They found that 23 of 75 patients with primary HS virus infections had significant increases in complement-fixing antibody to varicella virus. In tests on 42 patients with chickenpox-zoster infections (the two clinical entities were not distinguished), 5 had rises in complement-fixing antibody to HS virus. In both series, the rise in the titre of antibody to the heterologous virus occurred only in those with serological evidence of prior infection with that virus. The HS virus-infected patients who had a rise in titre of varicella virus complement-fixing antibody also had marked increases in varicella virus neutralizing antibody and antibody demonstrable by the immunofluorescence technique. Conversely, none of the chickenpox-zoster patients who developed heterologous complement-fixing antibody increases developed corresponding increases in the titre of neutralizing antibody to HS virus, and in only one was a 4-fold increase in antibody demonstrable by the immunofluorescence technique. It appears, however, that all the HS cases were primary ones, while only 2 of the 5 chickenpox-zoster cases tested for neutralizing and fluorescent antibody were chickenpox cases and the only rise in fluorescent antibody titre occurred in one of these.

In summary, it appears that in complement-fixation tests with varicella or HS virus antigens produced from infected tissue-culture cells, significant rises in the titre of heterologous as well as homologous antibodies are likely to occur in the sera of patients suffering primary infections with either virus and who have had previous experience of the heterologous one. Patients who suffer recurrent HS virus infections and zoster patients are less likely to exhibit this heterologous response. Primary infection with HS virus may also elicit marked increases in varicella virus neutralizing antibody and in antibody demonstrable by immunofluorescence in subjects who have had prior experience of varicella virus. The reciprocal response in chickenpox patients does not seem to occur. It is likely, therefore, that some common antigen or antigens occur in varicella and HS viruses. These cross-reactions have been demonstrated only with human sera, however, and do not seem to occur with hyper-immune sera produced experimentally in animals. It can be argued, therefore, that they may respresent a lack of specificity of the early antibodies rather than the sharing of antigens. Some preliminary investigations into the antigenic relationship between varicella and HS viruses using the gel-diffusion technique have been described by TRLIFAJOVÁ et al. (1970) who used antigens prepared by freezing and thawing concentrated suspensions of infected tissue-culture cells and human sera concentrated two-fold. They found that 2 sera, one from a convalescent zoster patient and the other from a blood donor, precipitated with both varicella and HS virus antigens and that one precipitation line was common to the two antigens; that is, there was a reaction of partial identity probably due to a shared common antigen.

KRECH and JUNG (1971) reported that infants and children with cytomegalic inclusion disease demonstrable by virus isolation or by a complement-fixing antibody response did not have a complement-fixing antibody response to varicella virus. Apart from this report, however, the possible antigenic relationship of varicella virus to other members of the herpesvirus group has not been reported.

V. Cultivation

A. Growth in Tissue-Culture Cells

1. Susceptibility of Various Cell Types

Almost all those who have studied varicella virus have used monolayer (or explant) tissue cultures. WELLER and STODDARD (1952), however, first demonstrated cytopathic changes (intranuclear inclusions) in suspended tissue fragments

Table 3. *Tissue Cultures Susceptible to Varicella Virus*

Cell Cultures[1]	References to virus effect
PRIMARY	
H. E. skin muscle fibroblasts	WELLER (1953), WELLER et al. (1958), TAYLOR-ROBINSON (1959), GURVICH (1962)
H. E. lung fibroblasts	RAPP and BENYESH-MELNICK (1963), MEURISSE (1969)
H. E. fibroblasts (whole embryo)	TOURNIER et al. (1957), GÉDER et al. (1963), GÉDER et al. (1964)
Human foreskin fibroblasts	WELLER (1953), WELLER et al. (1958), TAYLOR-ROBINSON (1959)
Human kidney	WELLER et al. (1958), GOLD (1965)
Human amnion	WELLER et al. (1958), TAYLOR-ROBINSON (1959), ROSANOFF (1963), CAUNT and TAYLOR-ROBINSON (1964), NETTER (1964), GOLD (1965), SCHMIDT et al. (1965), MEURISSE (1969)
Human thyroid	CAUNT (1963), CAUNT and TAYLOR-ROBINSON (1964), GÉDER et al. (1964), GOLD (1965), MEURISSE (1969)
Rhesus monkey kidney	WELLER et al. (1958), ROSANOFF (1963), GÉDER et al. (1964), SCHMIDT et al. (1965 a), SCHMIDT et al. (1965 b), MEURISSE (1969)
African green monkey kidney	ROSANOFF (1963), SLOTNICK and ROSANOFF (1963), MEURISSE (1969)
Baboon kidney	ROSANOFF (1963)
Rabbit kidney	WELLER et al. (1958)
Guinea pig embryo fibroblasts	SÖLTZ-SZÖTS (1964; 1965)
DIPLOID	
H. E. skin muscle	ROSANOFF (1963), SCHMIDT et al. (1964)
H. E. lung	ROSANOFF (1963), SLOTNICK and ROSANOFF (1963), KAPSENBERG (1964), BRUNELL (1967b), SCHMIDT et al. (1969)
H. E. kidney	SCHMIDT et al. (1965 a; 1965 b)
WI-38 (H. E. lung) (HAYFLICK and MOORHEAD, 1961)	ROSANOFF (1963), RAWLS et al. (1964), HERRMANN (1967), MARTOS et al. (1970)
Human placental fibroblasts (RAWLS and HERRMANN, 1964)	RAWLS et al. (1964), HERRMANN (1967)
Human foreskin fibroblasts	KISSLING et al. (1968)
CONTINUOUS	
HeLa (GEY et al., 1952)	WELLER et al. (1958), GOLD (1965), SVEDMYR (1965), MEURISSE (1969)
Human amnion F. L. (FOGH and LUND, 1957)	ROSANOFF (1963)
BS-C-1 (African green monkey kidney) (HOPPS et al., 1963)	ROSANOFF (1963), SLOTNICK and ROSANOFF (1963)
GMK-AH-1 (Grivet monkey kidney) (GUNALP, 1965)	SVEDMYR (1966), KISSLING et al. (1968)
VERO (Vervet monkey kidney) (LIEBHABER et al., 1967)	CAUNT and SHAW (1969), TAWARA and OGIWARA (1969)
V 3 A (Vervet monkey kidney) (BEALE and CHRISTOFINIS, 1964)	MEURISSE (1969)
Monkey kidney III/I (RUZICSKA, 1964)	GÉDER et al. (1964)

H. E. = human embryo.   [1] References in this column to first description of cell culture.

of human embryos of 2—3 months gestation and noted that the virus could not be subcultured by transfer of fluid from such infected cultures. Later, WELLER (1953) showed that the virus could be propagated serially in human fibroblast cultures only if intact, infected cells were subcultured to fresh tissue cultures. In an extensive study, WELLER et al. (1958) reported the isolation of varicella virus in tissue cultures of human embryo skin-muscle, human fore-skin and adult human uterus and testis. They subcultured virus in these tissues and also in human embryo brain, human post-natal kidney, human amnion, HeLa cells, and in rhesus monkey kidney and testis cultures. They had also some evidence for transfer of infection to rabbit testis and kidney cell cultures but the infection was rapidly lost on serial transfer in these tissue cells. Their attempts to grow virus in chick tissues, murine and bovine embryo tissues and porcine kidney cells were not successful. Subsequent work has confirmed that isolation and serial cultivation of varicella virus can be achieved only in tissues of human or primate origin and that in most cases virus remains cell-associated. Most investigators have used either human embryo fibroblast cultures or human amnion cells but other primary and continuous cultures of human and simian cells have been used, as shown in Table 3. ROSANOFF (1963) noted that among the cell types he used, the highest yield of infected cells was obtained from human embryo lung diploid fibroblasts (including WI-38 cells) or primary African green monkey kidney cells, and that the continuous lines of 'FL' human amnion cells or 'BS-C-1' African green monkey kidney cells were preferable to primary rhesus or baboon kidney cells.

CAUNT (1963) showed (see p. 30) that infectious virus could be liberated in a cell-free state following ultrasonic disruption of primary cultures of human thyroid cells, a finding which was confirmed by GÉDER et al. (1964) and by GOLD (1965). Cell-free virus has been liberated also from infected cultures of a continuous line of monkey kidney cells by GÉDER et al. (1964), from human embryo lung fibroblasts by BRUNELL (1967 b) and from primary cultures of baboon thyroid cells by SHAW (1968). The isolation of virus and spontaneous release of cell-free infectious virus in primary cultures of guinea pig embryo tissues has been reported by SÖLTZ-SZÖTS (1964, 1965) but does not appear to have been investigated or confirmed by other workers.

GÉDER et al. (1965) produced a persistent varicella virus infection in the continuous line of III/I monkey kidney cells. The infection persisted through ten subcultures of the cells with alternating periods of cell destruction and regrowth.

Little information is available about the relative sensitivity of the various cell cultures used for virus isolation. CAUNT and TAYLOR-ROBINSON (1964) noted that primary cultures of human thyroid cells were more sensitive than primary cultures of human amnion for virus isolation and MEURISSE (1969) isolated virus more frequently in human thyroid than in human amnion cells. SCHMIDT et al. (1965 a) noted that human foetal diploid kidney cells appeared to be as sensitive for virus isolation as similar cells in primary culture and more sensitive than primary cultures of rhesus monkey kidney or human amnion cells. HERRMAN (1967) did not observe cytopathic changes in primary cultures of rhesus monkey kidney cells or HeLa cells inoculated with chickenpox vesicle fluid from which virus could be isolated in human foetal diploid fibroblasts. GÉDER et al. (1963) had previously failed to isolate or propagate the virus in HeLa cells although WELLER et al. (1958)

had used this cell line to maintain virus strains and SVEDMYR (1965) used it for virus isolation and propagation. Perhaps this reflects differences in the susceptibility to varicella virus of different strains of HeLa cells in use in various laboratories. Variation in the sensitivity of HeLa cells to other viruses is known to exist. Alternatively WELLER (1969) suggests that the apparent insusceptibility of some HeLa cells to varicella virus may be due to the use of poor maintenance medium in which growth of cells ceases and development of virus may consequently be poor or negligible. Inhibition of varicella virus multiplication by mycoplasmas contaminating the cell cultures is a possibility that has not been investigated.

2. Cytopathogenicity

In unfixed cell culture, infection is first detectable as areas of increased refractility of groups of cells and especially their nuclei, which are readily visible by phase contrast and even by direct light microscopy, 2 days or more after inocula-

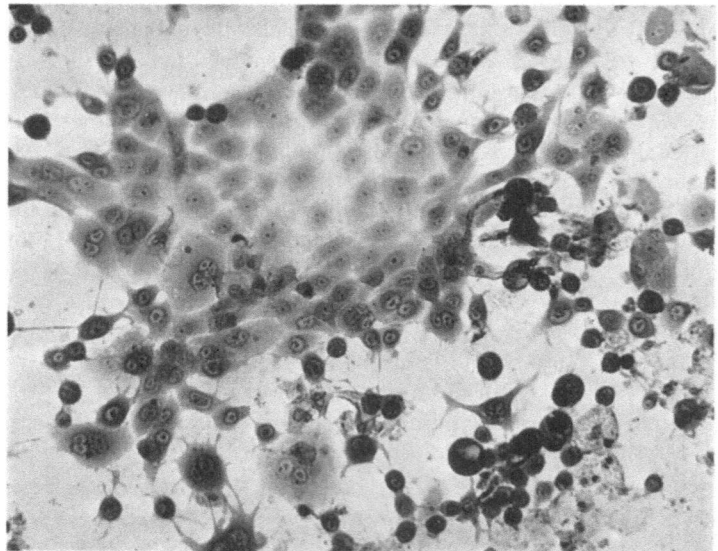

Fig. 2. Cytopathic effect in human amnion cells produced by varicella virus from zoster vesicle fluid. The changes are the same as those produced by virus from chickenpox vesicle fluid. × 150

tion. The earliest cytopathic effect recorded is 1 day after inoculation of primary human thyroid cells (MEURISSE, 1969) and the latest is 21 days after inoculation of primary human amnion cells (GOLD, 1965). Later the cells become rounded, swollen and separated from one another (Fig. 2) and eventually become detached from the glass (WELLER, 1953); see also Fig. 8. Frequently multinucleate giant cells develop (Fig. 3). The tendency to form such cells seems to vary with the tissue used for cultivation, the passage history of the virus and the amount of virus inoculated, always being greatest with a high dose of infective material. Their presence may, however, be the result of heterogeneity of the virus since two distinct variants of a strain isolated from zoster have been described by NII and

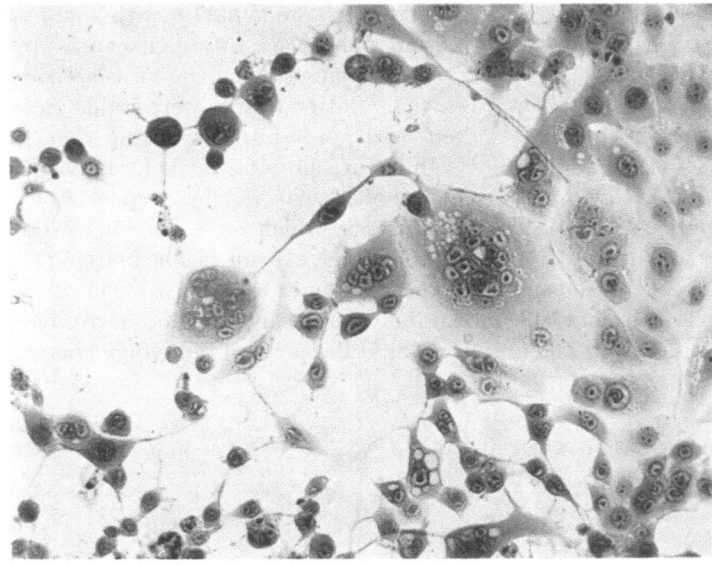

Fig. 3. Multinucleated giant cells, each nucleus containing an inclusion body, in an amnion cell culture inoculated with chickenpox vesicle fluid. × 190. From D. Taylor-Robinson, Brit. J. exp. Path., **40**, 521—532 (1959)

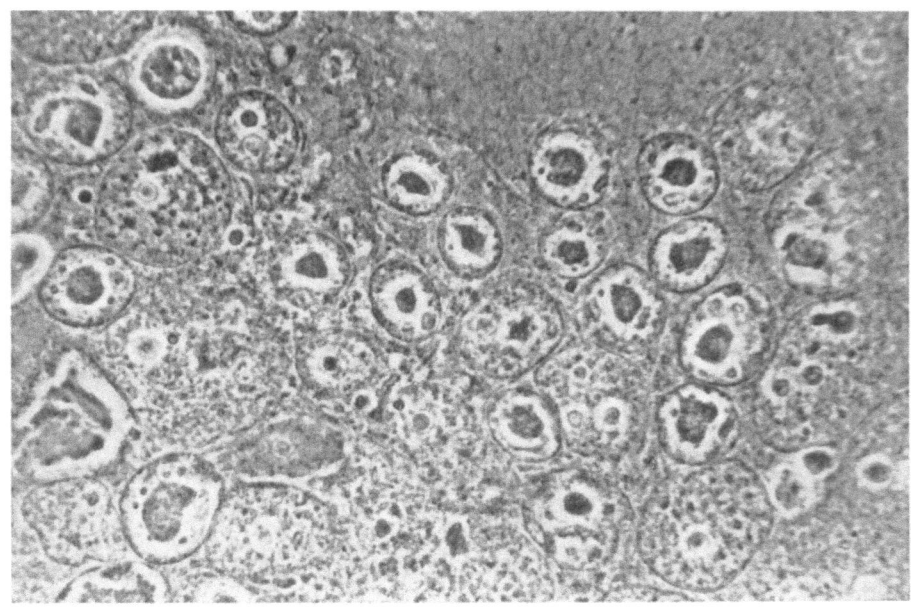

Fig. 4. Nuclei in a syncytium formed by He La cells infected with varicella virus. Fixed in absolute alcohol, observed by phase contrast microscopy and photographed unstained. × 1000. Note the inclusion body separated from the marginal chromatin by a clear halo. From J. S. F. Niven (1961)

MAEDA (1969). One variant gave rise to large syncytia with rapid spread of the virus throughout the culture, while the other, although causing characteristic rounding-up of the cells, produced few syncytia and the virus spread more slowly and the foci of infection were smaller. Both variants were stable on subculture.

In infected cultures treated with protein-precipitating fixatives such as Zenker's, Bouin's and Carnoy's fluids or absolute alcohol, many of the cells are seen to contain intranuclear inclusions, separated by a space from the nuclear membrane (see Fig. 4). These inclusions, which have a strong affinity for eosin especially in cultures fixed in Zenker's fluid, are not visible in living cells examined by phase contrast microscopy, nor are they in cells fixed for electron microscopy in Palade's solution which contains 1 per cent osmium tetroxide buffered to pH 7.4 (see Fig. 5). The only striking differences at this stage compared with the

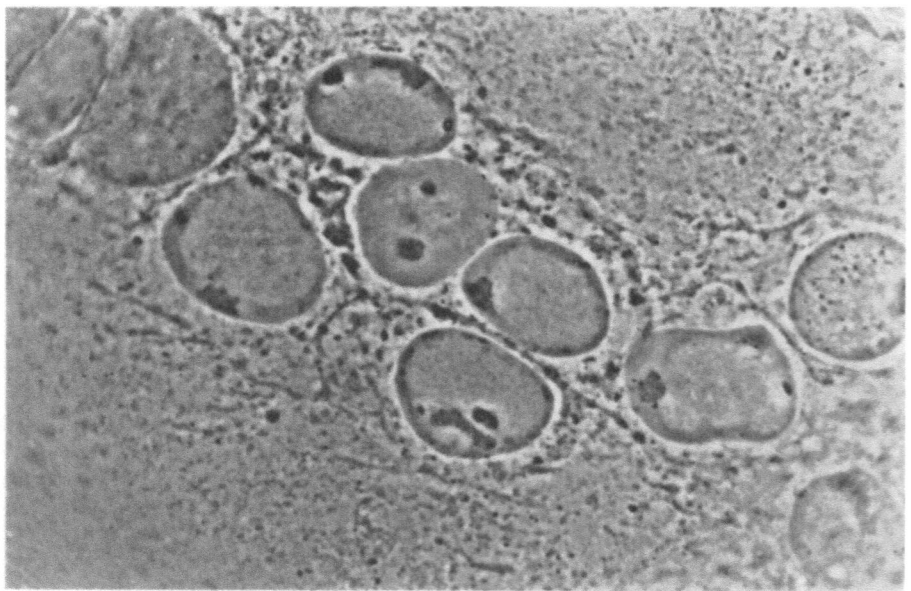

Fig. 5. Nuclei of HeLa cells infected with varicella virus. Fixed in Palade's solution (1 per cent osmium tetroxide, pH 7.4), observed by phase contrast microscopy and photographed unstained. × 1460. Margination of chromatin is visible but inclusion bodies have not developed. From J. S. F. NIVEN (1961)

nuclei of uninfected cells are in increased nuclear size, increased peripheral density on the inner side of the nuclear membrane due to DNA, confirmed by the Feulgen reaction, and an increase in size and alteration in shape of the nucleoli which often assume a peripheral localization. The intranuclear inclusion may be regarded therefore as a phenomenon observed when certain types of commonly-used protein-precipitating fixatives are used (see pp. 25 and 32). It has also been observed that before inclusion bodies can be demonstrated by fixation, small basophilic chromatin granules are seen to be widely distributed throughout the nucleoplasm and it is this material which apparently becomes displaced towards the nuclear membrane as the inclusion substance develops.

The avidity of the inclusions for acidophilic stains such as eosin has already been mentioned and they can be shown also to be Feulgen negative. In infected cultures fixed in alcohol or Carnoy's fluid, stained with acridine orange (ARMSTRONG and NIVEN, 1957) and examined by fluorescence microscopy with blue-violet light (400—450 mμ), typical inclusions emit a dull greenish fluorescence which contrasts with the greenish-yellow fluorescence given by the Feulgen-positive DNA accumulations close to the nuclear membrane. This dull green fluorescence is not removed by alcohol treatment but is completely removed by pepsin (2 mg/ml) digestion, while the nuclear DNA remains unaffected, as shown by its Feulgen-positive reaction. Short wave ultraviolet microscopy of the inclusions has revealed a maximum absorption at 275 mμ, that of the nucleic acid material being at 257 mμ. The DNA localized in the neighbourhood of the nuclear membrane can be removed by 0.005 per cent DNase in veronal acetate buffer containing magnesium ions. This indicates that it is probably not mature virus, which is often DNase resistant: electron microscope observations (ARMSTRONG, J. A., personal communication) confirm this finding.

Fluorescent antibody studies (see p. 31) indicate that the mature inclusion does not contain virus structural antigens, while the results of auto-radiographic studies (see p. 32) suggest that the inclusion is the site of viral DNA synthesis although this synthesis is mainly completed before the eosinophilic inclusion is demonstrable. Thus the inclusion may be regarded as precipitated abnormal protein residues found during and remaining after the intranuclear phase of virus synthesis (see p. 32). The exact chemical nature of the residues remains uncertain.

Several investigators have used the electron microscope to follow the replication of varicella virus in tissue-culture cells. A variety of cell systems has been used and it may not always be possible to compare the results of one study with those of another. The work of TOURNIER et al. (1957) has been mentioned already (p. 8). They described the development of virus particles in human embryo fibroblasts. The earliest particles occurred in the nucleus of infected cells and there was progression from granularity in the nucleus to distinct particles with a dense central body surrounded by a single membrane. Particles in the cytoplasm and outside the cells had two membranes and resembled particles in vesicle fluid. In the cytoplasm the particles were often present inside large membrane-bounded vacuoles. In spite of finding apparently mature particles outside the cells, infection could not be transmitted by cell-free tissue-culture fluid.

BECKER et al. (1965) used human embryo fibroblast cultures to compare the development of varicella virus isolated from zoster with that of human cytomegalovirus, another cell-associated herpesvirus. They found that virus "cores" with a single membrane were formed in the nucleus and that they appeared to acquire a second coat on passage through the nuclear membrane. In the cytoplasm virus particles were often located within irregular membrane-bound vesicles, possibly formed by the endo-plasmic reticulum. In the vesicles some of the particles acquired additional coats, but they did not seem to receive extra layers on passage through the plasma membrane which remained intact after the virus had left the cell. The virus particles varied in size according to the number of layers they had acquired. Extra-cellular virus was pleomorphic and many particles seemed to be devoid of a central core or nucleoid while others had a single coat only.

Similar observations were reported by ACHONG and MEURISSE (1968) who studied human amnion cells infected with varicella virus. Particles with a single membrane were found in the nucleus and the cytoplasm and these particles acquired a second coat either on passage through the nuclear membrane, or on passing into cytoplasmic vacuoles, or at the plasmalemma. Thus, double-coated particles were found in the perinuclear space, within the cytoplasm and also outside the cell where they were closely associated with the cell surface. In spite of large numbers of morphologically mature particles outside the cell, again, no cell-free infectious virus could be demonstrated. They suggested that varicella virus is functionally deficient although apparently morphologically complete.

COOK and STEVENS (1968), however, attribute the lack of infectivity of varicella virus to the lability of its coat. In detailed studies (COOK and STEVENS, 1968; 1970) of the growth of varicella virus in human amnion cells they found full, double-coated particles present near the nuclear membrane but inside the nucleus. They also found "naked" capsids inside the nucleus sometimes in crystalline array, but these did not have a dense central core although they sometimes contained a ring-like structure. Virus particles were observed budding through the nuclear membrane and the outer layer of the virion appeared to be continuous with the inner nuclear membrane. Virus particles were never observed budding from the plasma membrane or receiving envelope material from any cytoplasmic structures. Indeed, when the mature double-coated particles passed to the cytoplasm they tended to become pleomorphic and displayed open envelopes, disrupted capsids and a paucity of dense central cores. Outside the cell these bizarre forms were even more evident. COOK and STEVENS suggest that the virus is synthesized in the nucleus complete with core and double membrane, but outside the nucleus the virus coat is disrupted with consequent loss of the core and of infectivity. These workers reported that 26 per cent of the particles in the nucleus had cores, but only 9 per cent of the extracellular particles did so and many had broken coats or capsids. Different results were reported by SHAW (1968) who examined a virus suspension prepared by ultrasonic disruption of infected human thyroid cells. This suspension contained 10^5 p.f.u./ml but 8×10^{10} total particles of which 18 per cent were full (dense central cores) and were enveloped (double coated), 7 per cent were empty and enveloped, 70 per cent were full and not enveloped and 5 per cent were empty and not enveloped. This is in marked contrast to the observations of COOK and STEVENS (1968) who found that only 9 per cent of extracellular particles were full. Even so, if it is assumed that a virus particle needs to be full and enveloped to be infectious, Shaw's preparation had 1.4×10^{10}/ml of such particles but only 10^5 infectious units could be demonstrated. It thus seems likely that while morphological integrity may be essential for infectivity additional factors are concerned.

These electron microscope studies have been carried out in a variety of cell systems and the processes described may not be strictly comparable.

Chromosomal changes. BENYESH-MELNICK et al. (1964) observed chromosomal aberrations in primary cultures of human embryo lung diploid fibroblasts infected with varicella virus from a zoster case. The normal mitotic cycle was arrested in metaphase and many of the chromosomes were over-contracted and scattered throughout the cells. Chromosomes of many cells, however, were eventually able to uncoil and enter interphase without anaphasic movement with the result that micronuclei of varying sizes were formed. The mitotic arrest in metaphase and asynchronous entrance into interphase are similar to the effects of colchicine on normal cells in tissue culture. Chromatid and chromosome breakage was observed in many metaphase plates of infected cultures. In 4 samples taken 24 hours after infection, chromatid and chromosome breaks ranged from 26 per cent to 45 per cent compared to 2.1 per cent in the control uninfected cultures. Chromosome fragmentation occurred in 68 per cent to 81 per cent of the blocked metaphase plates although some of the fragments may have represented uncoiled chromosomes still connected by fibrous structures.

The significance of these findings in studies of infected tissue-culture cells is not known, but they are of interest in view of the conflicting evidence concerning chromosomal abnormalities in leukocytes of patients with chickenpox (p. 45).

3. Plaque Formation

Cytopathic changes in tissue-culture monolayers are first observable about 2 days after infection as foci of cells with increased refractility. As infection progresses the cells become rounded and tend to separate, leaving long fine strands

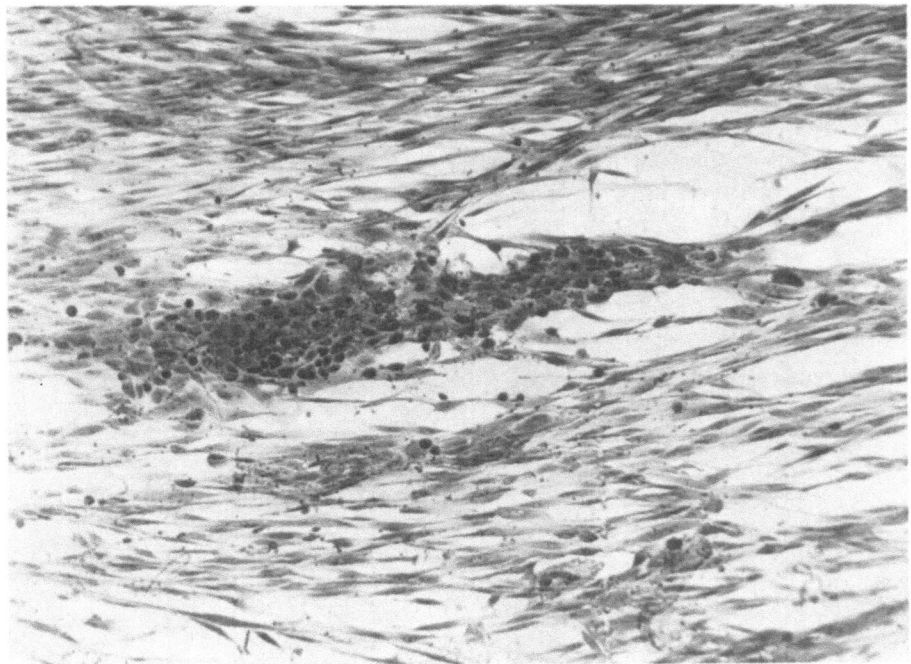

Fig. 6. A microplaque in a monolayer of human fibroblasts produced by varicella virus from zoster vesicle fluid
× 90

of cytoplasm connecting one cell with another. These microplaques (Figs. 6 and 7) can be counted under a low-power microscope (× 10 to × 40 magnification) after 4—8 days, depending on the type of cells used (WELLER et al., 1958; TAYLOR-ROBINSON, 1959; CAUNT and SHAW, 1969). The initial foci of infection extend by the involvement of contiguous cells and the earliest infected cells at the centre die

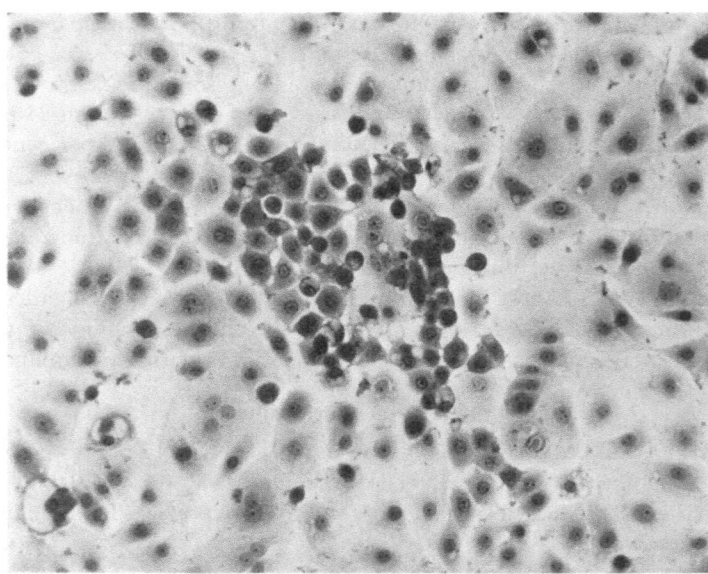

Fig. 7. A microplaque in a monolayer of human amnion cells produced by varicella virus from chickenpox vesicle fluid. × 150

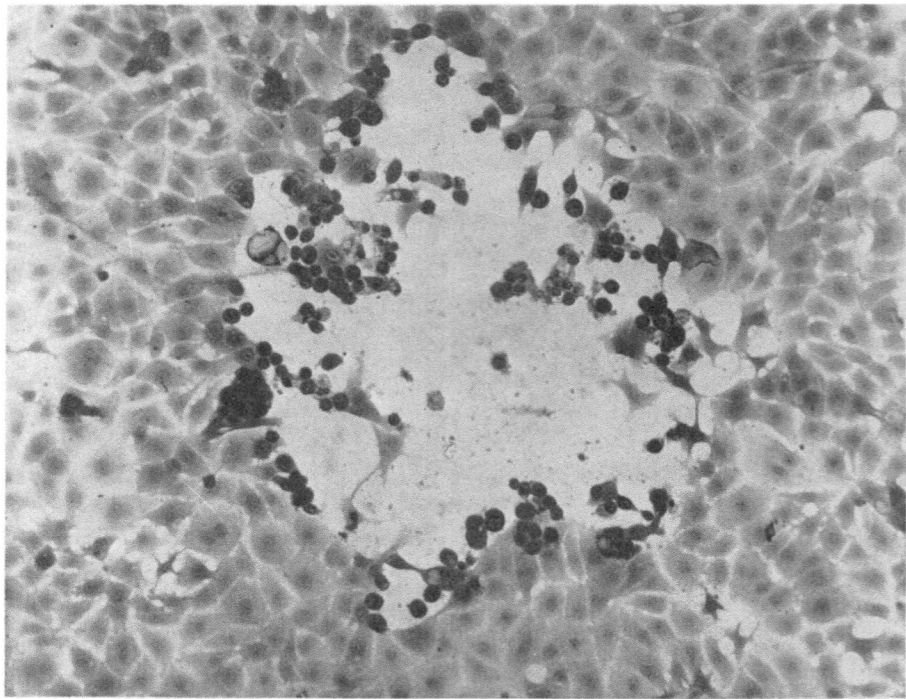

Fig. 8. A focal lesion in a monolayer of human amnion cells produced by varicella virus. The degenerate cells in the centre have fallen off the glass. × 180

and fall off the glass (Fig. 8). In this way macroplaques are formed which can be counted by the naked eye (Fig. 9). These plaques continue to increase in size but do not usually increase in number, except in a few tissues from which infectious virus is spontaneously released, *e.g.* human thyroid cells. RAPP and BENYESH-MELNICK (1963), however, found that satisfactory plaque counts in human embryo lung fibroblasts could be achieved only if an agar overlay was used, presumably because secondary plaques were initiated by dislodgement of infected

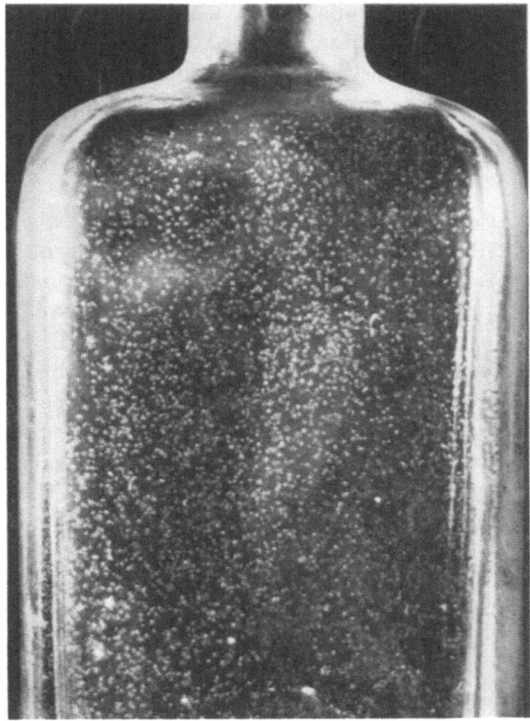

Fig. 9. A flat surfaced glass bottle containing a monolayer of human amnion cells that had been inoculated 15 days previously with a suspension of varicella virus-infected amnion cells. Plaques of infected cells are visible

cells in cultures with a fluid overlay. The addition of neutral red to the agar overlay allowed plaques to be counted as soon as the infected cells died and excluded the dye. This happens earlier than detachment of cells from the glass to form macroplaques under liquid overlay. ROSANOFF (1963) used a similar technique to produce plaques, visible to the naked eye, in human diploid fibroblasts and African green monkey kidney cells.

4. Virus Multiplication

a) Adsorption of Virus to Cells

Cell-free virus appears to adsorb slowly to tissue-culture cells. CAUNT and TAYLOR-ROBINSON (1964) found that only about half the virus in vesicle fluid was adsorbed to human amnion or thyroid cells after incubation at 37° C for 3 hours and that maximum adsorption required 9—12 hours. Similar results were obtained using virus prepared from infected human thyroid cells.

In contrast, infected cells in suspension appear to transmit infection to fresh cells much more rapidly. RAPP (1964) produced plaques by using infected human embryo fibroblasts as inoculum and overlaying the cell sheet with agar before incubation. He found that removal of the inoculum of infected cells after 15 minutes' contact with a fresh cell sheet did not reduce the number of plaques which subsequently developed. He also showed no significant increase in the number of plaques when the adsorption period was increased from 15 to 240 minutes. Similarly, GOLD (1965) found that at 30° to 40° C transfer of infection from an inoculum of cells was almost complete in 30 minutes or less, but noted that at 25° C and 4° C transfer was slower, requiring 1 to 2 hours, and that the plaque counts were 50 per cent and 10 per cent, respectively, of those achieved at 37° C.

b) Effect of Temperature

WELLER et al. (1958) observed that the cytopathic effect of varicella virus in human fibroblast cultures progressed much more slowly at 25° C than at 35° C. The effect of temperature on the growth of the virus in primary cultures of human embryo fibroblasts was further investigated by VÁCZI et al. (1963). They found that growth was most rapid and the yield of infected cells maximal at 37° C. At 30° C the rate of growth was much reduced although ultimately the yield was as great as at 37° C. This slower virus multiplication reflects perhaps the much slower growth of the tissue cultures at 30° C. At 39° C cytopathic effects were not seen in most experiments but when they did occur infected cells died and became detached from the glass leaving only healthy, non-infectious cells in the culture. While virus growth did not occur at 39° C, infected tissue cultures kept at this temperature for up to one week were still capable on subsequent transfer to 37° C of yielding infectious cells and cytopathic effects were then detected. Similar results were obtained by GOLD (1965) who studied infected human amnion cells. He found also that the maximum yield of infected cells was obtained at 37° C but that comparable yields were obtained after incubation for 1 week at 24° C or 30° C followed by 1 week at 37° C. However, incubation for 1 week at 40° C resulted in complete loss of virus in the cells.

c) Production of Cell-Free Virus

Cell-free virus can be obtained by suitable treatment of various cell cultures (see p. 21). If human thyroid cells are disrupted by ultrasonic vibration at various intervals after infection no free virus is found up to 24 hours, but it is detectable at 36 hours and reaches its maximum at 48 to 72 hours (CAUNT, 1967). At this time intranuclear inclusions can be demonstrated in the cells but no gross cytopathic changes are evident. If at 48 to 72 hours the infected thyroid cells from a monolayer of 84 sq. cm. (cells on one side of a 12 oz. medical prescription bottle) are disrupted in a volume of 2 ml, a cell-free virus suspension with a titre of 10^5 p.f.u./ml may be obtained (CAUNT and TAYLOR-ROBINSON, 1964). Infectious virus also appears spontaneously in the supernatant medium of the cell culture about 48 hours after infection, but it rarely exceeds 100 p.f.u./ml even after 96 hours (CAUNT, unpublished). CAUNT and TAYLOR-ROBINSON (1964) showed also that the number of plaque-forming units of free virus obtained by ultrasonic disruption of cells was only about 10 per cent of the number of plaque-forming infected cells from which it was prepared. Undoubtedly most of the virus released by this treatment is non-infectious (see SHAW, 1968; quoted in the section on cytopathogenicity).

BRUNELL (1967 b) obtained cell-free virus by disrupting with ultrasonic vibration human embryo lung fibroblasts 3 days after they had been infected and when 70 per cent of the cell monolayer showed cytopathic changes. He treated the cells from a 32 oz. prescription bottle in 2 ml of medium and obtained cell-free virus preparations with infectivity titres of 1.1×10^4 to 1.4×10^5 p.f.u./ml. This was less (12.5 per cent to 72 per cent) than the number of infected cells in the original suspension. He also noted that if the infected cells were removed from the glass with trypsin instead of versene the yield of infectious virus subsequently obtained was markedly diminished. This effect of trypsin was confirmed by SHAW (1968) using human thyroid cell cultures. It is possible that the failure to demonstrate infectious cell-free virus in some other types of infected cell cultures may be due to the use of trypsin for removing the cells from the glass rather than their inherent inability to produce such virus. This is not the whole answer, however, because SVEDMYR (1965) failed to obtain free virus from HeLa cells which were removed from the glass with versene.

GÉDER et al. (1964/65) used trypsin to remove their infected cell monolayers from the glass and treated the cells with ultrasonic vibration for 10 minutes to liberate virus from them. From 100 sq. cm of cells of a continuous line of monkey kidney or a primary culture of human thyroid they obtained a total yield of $3—4 \times 10^2$ p.f.u. of cell-free infectious virus. They also found that 50—100 p.f.u./ml of virus were released spontaneously into the supernatant fluids from these cultures.

SHAW (1968) found that primary cultures of baboon thyroid cells gave the same final yield of cell-free virus as human thyroid cells but he did not investigate the complete growth cycle in baboon cells.

d) Detection of Viral Antigen by Immunofluorescence

WELLER and COONS (1954) first demonstrated that cells infected with varicella virus could be detected by the immunofluorescence technique using convalescent sera from chickenpox or zoster patients. Since then various investigators have used this method to demonstrate the position and spread of varicella virus within infected cells. SLOTNICK and ROSANOFF (1963) described the appearance of varicella virus antigen in BS-C-1 cells, a continuous line of African green monkey kidney cells (HOPPS et al., 1963). A perinuclear fluorescence developed, first visible at 24 hours but much more pronounced at 48 to 72 hours after infection. Many of the infected cells were swollen and contained fluorescent granules in their cytoplasm at 72 hours and by 96 hours the cells were much smaller and the fluorescence was reduced to faint blobs. The sequence of events in primary cultures of African green monkey kidney cells and in a diploid strain of human embryo lung fibroblasts was similar except that antigen appeared earlier.

RAPP and VANDERSLICE (1964) compared the spread of varicella virus antigen in human embryo lung fibroblasts with the increase in number of cells capable of initiating plaque formation. They found that up to 8 hours after infection there was no spread of virus from the cells initially infected, but by 16 hours the number of plaque-forming cells had at least doubled and foci of 1 to 6 fluorescent cells were observed. By 40 hours after inoculation about 50 per cent of the cells in the cell sheet were infected, representing about 15 infected cells for every infectious cell in the inoculum. They noted that antigen was often observed in the nuclei but appeared to predominate in the cytoplasm. Large round cells containing virus antigen were observed 32 hours after infection, at the same time that cytopathic effects were first noted in the cultures.

In similar studies by KOLLER et al. (1963), virus antigen was detected in the nuclei of infected cells 10 hours after infection, progressed to fill the nuclei by 24 to 48 hours, and after 24 hours it was present in the cytoplasm as well. Nuclear fluorescence diminished after 48 hours and by 144 hours practically disappeared although there was still specific fluorescence in the cytoplasm. They tried to relate these changes to the cytopathic effects demonstrated by haematoxylin and eosin staining and their results suggest that the intranuclear eosinophilic inclusions appear at a time when virus antigen is diminishing in the nucleus. It is difficult to equate these last findings with those of RAPP and VANDERSLICE (1964) or SLOT-NICK and ROSANOFF (1963) whose results did not suggest the presence of large amounts of antigen in the nucleus of infected cells. However, from a consideration of all these results it seems likely that the earliest appearance of varicella virus antigen (presumably virus structural protein) is about 10 hours after inoculation of a culture with infected cells. A likely sequence of events is that virus nucleic acid is transferred from infected to non-infected cells within 30 minutes of their contact (p. 30) and that 10 hours elapse before virus antigen formation becomes apparent. Antigen production is at its maximum about 40 hours after infection and subsequently diminishes, possibly as the antigen is assembled into virus particles which then leave the cells.

e) DNA Synthesis in Infected Cells

NII and MAEDA (1970) investigated the incorporation of H^3-thymidine into Vero cells infected with varicella virus. They found that if infected cells were incubated in the presence of the H^3-thymidine the areas of the nucleus where eosinophilic inclusions were present became heavily labelled with the isotope while the remainder of the nucleus did not, suggesting that host cell DNA synthesis had ceased in infected cells but that viral DNA synthesis incorporating the isotopically labelled thymidine was proceeding in the inclusion body area. In the reverse experiment using pre-labelled cells which were then infected in the absence of isotope, the inclusion areas were free of isotope while the host cell DNA at the periphery of the nucleus was heavily labelled. If pre-labelled but uninfected cells were mixed with unlabelled infected ones and incubated in the absence of label then the first signs of infection in the labelled cells occurred at 16 hours when areas less densely labelled were visible in the nucleus. Small eosinophilic inclusions were demonstrable by 19 hours and these coincided with areas which were lacking in isotopic label. By 24 hours the inclusions almost filled the nucleus and it is suggested that the development of inclusion bodies is complete in 24—38 hours. The inclusion is thus probably the site of viral DNA synthesis although much of this synthesis occurs before the inclusion becomes demonstrable by fixation and staining with eosin (see pp. 24 and 25).

f) Interferon Production

WELLER *et al.* (1958) found no evidence that varicella virus-infected cultures of human fibroblasts produced any substance which interfered with the infection of normal cells of the cultures by herpes simplex virus. CAUNT and TAYLOR-ROBINSON (1964) also failed to demonstrate interferon production by primary human amnion or thyroid cells infected with varicella virus. GÉDER *et al.* (1965), however, using the III/I continuous line of monkey kidney cells chronically infected with varicella virus found that the culture fluid, concentrated 10 times, contained a substance capable of inhibiting the growth of vaccinia virus. The concentrated culture fluid was incubated with non-infected III/I cells for 24 hours and then removed before the vaccinia inoculum was added. The subsequent plaque count of vaccinia virus was reduced about 50 per cent by this treatment.

Interferon has been found by WHEELOCK (1967) in the crusts from chickenpox patients and in greater concentration in chickenpox vesicle fluids by ARMSTRONG *et al.* (1970). The latter authors also note that they have found varicella virus to be capable of stimulating the production of interferon in cultures of human cells and that the virus is moderately sensitive to the action of interferon (ARMSTRONG and MERIGAN, 1971). It is possible that interferon production provides an explanation for the interference phenomena noted by some workers during concurrent infections of chickenpox and measles (p. 40). Furthermore, ARMSTRONG *et al.* (1970) suggest that low levels of vesicular interferon early in the course of zoster may have a bearing on dissemination of the rash.

B. Growth in Cultures of Organized Tissue

The first successful attempt to grow varicella virus in the laboratory appears to have been that of GOODPASTURE and ANDERSON (1944) who inoculated fragments of adult human skin with zoster vesicle fluid and then grafted the fragments on to the chorio-allantoic membrane of 9 day-old chick embryos. The lesions produced in the skin did not vesiculate but otherwise resembled histologically those occurring in the natural disease. Intranuclear, eosinophilic inclusions occurred in the affected epithelial cells. The chick tissues were insusceptible to the virus.

BLANK *et al.* (1948) also grafted human fore-skin onto the chorioallantois and inoculated it 24 hours later with zoster vesicle fluid. After a further 6 days many of the infected skin cells contained intranuclear inclusion bodies. This work was repeated by CAUNT (1969) who infected human embryo lung and kidney grafts as well as skin and showed that the lesions resembled histologically those seen in the intact host. The infectious virus produced in these grafts was cell-free and it could be preserved, therefore, by storage at −70° C and neutralized completely with immune serum. In addition, similar organised tissue fragments were cultured satisfactorily by various *in vitro* methods and the virus which resulted from infecting these was cell-free also.

It is interesting that human embryo skin grown as organised tissue should be capable of supporting the growth of infectious cell-free virus while the same tissue grown in monolayer cultures produces mainly cell-associated virus.

C. Attempts to Grow Virus in Fertile Eggs

BURNET and LUSH (1936) recorded that varicella virus failed to grow in chick tissue in fertile eggs and this finding has been repeatedly observed by other workers (BUDDINGH, 1938; IRONS *et al.*, 1941; GOODPASTURE and ANDERSON, 1944). WELLER and STODDARD (1952) also failed to grow the virus by intra-amniotic inoculation of chick embryos with chickenpox vesicle fluid, although they did not mention whether this material was infectious for human tissue cultures.

There are, however, various reports in the literature on the growth of varicella virus in fertile eggs. It seems likely that some of these reports have been due to contamination of material with other viruses (TANIGUCHI *et al.*, 1935) and other reports (TEIXERIA, 1936 a and b; KIN, 1940; VASILENKO, 1966; VALLONE *et al.*, 1965 b; PATENKO, 1966) remain unconfirmed. Inoculation of chickenpox vesicle fluid onto the chorioallantois of 9 to 12 day-old fertile hens' eggs may result in the development of some areas of opacity, but these cannot be serially subcultured and the cells concerned do not show intranuclear inclusion bodies on histological examination.

VI. Experimental Hosts

Varicella virus appears to be extremely species specific and apart from man evidence of infection has been found only in vervet and green monkeys *(Cercopithecus lalandi* and *sabaeus)*. RIVERS (1926, 1927) inoculated young males of both species intratesticularly with emulsified vesicles and papules collected within 48 to 72 hours of the onset of the rash in chickenpox. In these animals spermatogenesis had not been initiated and he found intranuclear inclusions in cells in regions of the testes damaged by the inoculation. These inclusions were demonstrable 5 or 6 days after inoculation but not later than this (RIVERS, 1926). Subsequently (RIVERS, 1927), it was shown that intranuclear inclusions were not formed if the inoculum was mixed with convalescent-phase (14 to 21 days) chickenpox serum before it was injected, although the same material mixed with acutephase (3 days or less) serum still produced inclusions. Monkeys immunized by previous injections of varicella virus also failed to develop intranuclear inclusions on subsequent intratesticular inoculation.

ECKSTEIN (1933/34) inoculated monkeys intracerebrally with chickenpox or zoster vesicle fluids and reported that they died 4 to 5 weeks later with histological changes suggestive of encephalitis. MAGNUSSEN (1941) also claimed to have produced inflammatory changes in the monkey brain but neither his nor Eckstein's claim seem to have been investigated further.

RIVERS (1926) did not succeed in infecting other species of monkeys (rhesus, marmoset and S. American ringtail), rabbits, guinea pigs, rats and chickens. The earlier literature includes some reports of apparently successful transmission of varicella virus to common laboratory animals but these claims are carefully reviewed and largely discounted by COLE and KUTTNER (1925) who also record their own failure to infect rabbits, guinea pigs and rhesus monkeys by various routes and vervet monkeys by intradermal or intratesticular inoculation. They do not record the maturity of the vervet monkeys but they removed the testes for examination 1 to 4 days after inoculation and this, according to Rivers' results (RIVERS, 1926) would be too early to detect intranuclear inclusions in the cells.

The validity of the claim of REAGAN et al. (1953) to have infected monkeys (Cercopithecus sabaeus) has already been discussed (p. 8).

SEIDENBERG (1931) and NICOLAU and KOPIOWSKA (1938) distinguished the virus of zoster from herpes simplex virus by the inability of the former to infect the rabbit cornea. The reports, for example those of KIN (1939; 1940), of infection of animals with varicella virus almost certainly resulted from the accidental presence of herpes simplex virus in the inoculum or from infection with rabbit herpes viruses like Virus III of RIVERS and TILLETT (1923, 1924 a, b).

In none of the cases so far described was it possible to confirm the presence of varicella virus in the material used for inoculation, as monolayer tissue cultures were not then available. SHAW (1968) used varicella virus of known infectivity for tissue cultures to inoculate rabbits by corneal scarification and vervet (Cercopithecus pygerythrus), rhesus (Macaca mulatta), patas (Erythrocebus patas) and squirrel (Saimiri sciureus) monkeys by various routes. He did not succeed in producing signs of illness in the animals or any serological responses as judged by neutralization and complement-fixation tests. Male vervet monkeys were not used and, therefore, the work of RIVERS (1926, 1927) was not repeated.

HEUSCHELE (1960) described the occurrence of chickenpox in three young anthropoid apes, a chimpanzee, an orang-utan and a gorilla. The diagnosis was made on clinical grounds only, however, and subsequently GOLD (1966) reported that sera from the orang-utan during her convalescence did not contain complement-fixing antibody to varicella virus. It seems likely, therefore, that all three animals were infected with some other virus capable of producing a chickenpox-like illness in primates.

VII. Clinicopathological Features

Varicella virus causes disease of two clinical types: (i) chickenpox and (ii) zoster.

A. Chickenpox

1. Clinical Aspects

The incubation period ranges between 11 to 20 days, but is usually 13 to 17 days (GORDON and MEADER, 1929). Chickenpox acquired from persons with zoster has the same incubation period as that acquired from contact with patients with chickenpox (SIMPSON, 1952).

The occurrence of recognizable pre-eruptive symptoms is not a constant feature and in young children the appearance of the rash is often the first clinical event. However, in older children and adults headache, pains in the limbs, nausea or vomiting, pyrexia and erythematous rashes may occur for a period of about 24 hours before the specific rash appears. The commonest type of prodromal rash is scarlatiniform. Rarely, a morbilliform prodromal rash occurs.

The specific rash appears very rapidly without previous pain or itching. The lesions erupt in crops, each crop consisting of small, discrete, red macules or maculo-papules which, within a few hours, become clear vesicles. Each vesicle is superficial, being situated "on" rather than "in" the skin and is very often elliptical in outline, in contrast to those of smallpox which are round. The major axis of the ellipse runs parallel with the natural folds of the skin and never across. Most vesicles are unilocular. In a few hours skin organisms, chiefly staphylococci, invade the vesicle and the contents rapidly become purulent. The pustule so formed dries up in the course of 2 to 5 days forming a scab which separates after a variable interval, leaving a shallow pink cicatrix which later becomes white.

The earliest lesions of chickenpox are said to appear on the buccopharyngeal mucosa (HARRIES et al., 1951). The cutaneous eruption appears earliest and most profusely on the back and then on the chest and abdomen. The arms and legs are usually sparsely involved. In other words, the rash is centripetally disposed in contrast to the centrifugal distribution of the smallpox rash. Further, RICKETTS pointed out (quoted by HARRIES et al., 1951) that the lesions of chickenpox tend to occur in relatively greater profusion in concavities and protected parts than upon convexities and exposed surfaces, as is the case in smallpox. As the lesions occur usually in successive crops at intervals of a few days, the patient after some days has concurrently papules, vesicles, pustules and, possibly, scabs on the same area of skin. An abortive rash, proceeding no further than the vesicular or even papular stage, may occur occasionally. Only rarely does the rash become confluent, bullous or gangrenous. Occasionally, haemorrhage occurs in the eruption but then usually in persons being treated with immunosuppressive drugs and/or suffering from leukaemia or Hodgkin's disease (see p. 37).

In addition to the very early vesicles of the buccal mucosa, lesions may appear on the palpebral or ocular conjunctivae. In the former situation they do not cause trouble but on the ocular conjunctiva the disease may appear as a superficial phlyctenular keratitis due to vesiculation of the cornea (FRANDSEN, 1950; GRIFFIN and SEARLE, 1953), or as a deeper disciform keratitis. The former heals quickly with little scarring, while the latter may take six months to heal, leaving a large opacity.

The eruption is accompanied by a generalized lymphadenopathy, the sub-occipital and post-cervical glands being most noticeable as a result of secondarily infected scalp lesions.

2. Complications

a) Increased Severity

The severity of the disease varies from patient to patient, usually being most severe in infants and adults. If the rash appears between 5 and 10 days after birth the disease is more severe than if it occurs at an earlier age (EHRLICH et al., 1958) and indeed the deaths which have occurred have been in infants which have developed rashes during this period (RAINE, 1966). MARETIĆ and COORAY (1963) noted that in the tropical climate of Cyprus chickenpox was more severe with a greater proportion of deaths (COORAY, 1965) than in Yugoslavia. In addition, epidemics of chickenpox in a virgin population can have a high mortality rate; 19 per cent was recorded in French Equatorial Africa (MILLOUS, 1936). Some persons may have only a few scattered lesions and no systemic upset, while others may have a very profuse rash and be seriously ill, with temperatures ranging from

103° to 105° F. Pneumonitis may be severe in adults (HARPER *et al.*, 1969) and have a fatal outcome. The death rate among pregnant women with chickenpox pneumonia (44 per cent) is greater than among other adults (17 per cent) (PICKARD, 1968). RIGDON *et al.* (1962) reviewed fatal cases of chickenpox. YAMADA *et al.* (1968) reported a fatal chickenpox infection in a patient with hypogamma-globulinaemia, and particularly liable to develop a fulminating fatal illness are those patients who suffer from blood dyscrasias such as leukaemia (HOLBROOK, 1937; PINKEL, 1961). It should be emphasized, however, that the prognosis is not always serious and probably depends on the stage of the leukaemic process. For patients in remission, the risk is negligible; for those in relapse, chickenpox is more serious but can still have a favourable outcome (BODEY *et al.*, 1964). Those who are receiving massive steroid therapy and who develop chickenpox are, it seems, particularly prone to have severe disease (CHEATHAM *et al.*, 1956; HAGGERTY and ELEY, 1956; NICHOLS, 1957; FINKEL, 1961; ROSCHLAU, 1967). However, this may not always be so (FITZ and MEIKLEJOHN, 1956). FALLIERS and ELLIS (1965) and GIRSH *et al.* (1966) consider that the risk of death from chickenpox is relatively low in asthmatic patients receiving steroid therapy. Furthermore, FINE *et al.* (1969) record that a young boy on immunosuppressive therapy experienced an uneventful attack of chickenpox. HAYES *et al.* (1965) reported the fatal outcome of chickenpox in an adult patient with chronic active pulmonary tuberculosis. Patients with cartilage-hair hypoplasia, which is associated with a defect of cell-mediated immunity but normal serum immunoglobulin levels, tend to develop severe chickenpox infections (LUX *et al.*, 1970).

b) Involvement of Internal Organs

Complications of this kind are rare but the following have been observed: myocarditis (HACKEL, 1953) and pericarditis (MANDELBAUM and TERK, 1959), nephritis (BULLOWA and WISHIK, 1935; YUCEOGLU *et al.*, 1967), orchitis (WESSEL-HOEFT and PEARSON, 1950), myositis (EISENHOFF and MARCUS, 1958) and pneumonia. The latter has been observed as a complication of congenital chickenpox (BREWER, 1960) as well as in cases in young children (EISENKLAM, 1966) and adults (WARING *et al.*, 1942; TRIEBWASSER *et al.*, 1967). Pneumonia may lead to pulmonary calcification (MACKAY and CAIRNEY, 1960; KNYVETT, 1966). Compli-cations affecting the nervous system, either post-chickenpox polyneuritis (CHARLES, 1965; DAS and SAHA, 1965) or involvement of the central nervous system (SUZUKI *et al.*, 1967) have been described. However, their incidence is not high. In the general community, encephalitis has been estimated to occur about once in every 4,000 cases of chickenpox (KRUGMAN, 1960), an incidence greater than in measles. The occurrence in hospitalized patients is greater than this because the most severe cases go to hospital, but it is nevertheless infrequent. BULLOWA and WISHIK (1935) mention only 5 cases of encephalitis and 3 of meningitis seen in 2,534 patients over a 5-year period, and BOUGHTON (1966 a) saw acute meningo-encephalomyelitis in 38 of 1517 hospitalized patients. UNDERWOOD (1953) reviewed 120 published cases of nervous complication. Encephalitis comprised half of all the reported cases, cerebellar forms being typical of chickenpox encephalitis. The onset may be at any time between 3 days before and 20 days after the appearance of the rash, but it usually follows the eruption by 4 to 10 days. Death may occur (CHERNIAVSKAIA *et al.*, 1965). However, UNDERWOOD's series showed that only 10 per cent of cases died, 10 per cent being left with some permanent sequel and the remainder recovering.

c) Development of Zoster

Zoster may be regarded as a 'long-term' complication of chickenpox since it occurs usually years after the chickenpox infection. Occasionally, however, zoster occurs soon after the chickenpox eruption as an immediate complication. STOKES (1959) indicated that this was not an uncommon occurrence, but very few instances are recorded in the literature. ALLEN (1944) reported the occurrence of zoster 3 weeks after the onset of chickenpox in a 5-year-old boy. CHEATHAM *et al.* (1956) reported the case of a 4-year-old boy who, while undergoing immunosuppressive therapy, developed chickenpox and died 17 days later; at necropsy a zoster eruption was found on the abdomen and back. TAYLOR-ROBINSON (1960) recorded the case of an 8-year-old boy who developed cervical zoster 6 days after the onset of otherwise uncomplicated chickenpox.

3. Histopathological Changes

The specific microscopical features, which primarily affect the cell nucleus following infection with varicella virus, are similar in all tissues, although accompanying non-specific changes differ, depending on the tissue involved. In an area of infected cells various abnormalities of the cell nucleus are seen. The affected nuclei have marginated chromatin with the chromatin granules packed against the nuclear membrane. Within the nucleus there may be varying amounts of homogeneous basophilic material, or more often, depending on the maturity of the infectious process and on staining techniques, an eosinophilic rounded body encircled by a wide clear zone (COWDRY, 1934). The latter is the commonest form in section. Many nuclei enlarge, multinucleate giant cells may be seen with perhaps as many as 30 nuclei (UNNA, 1896), and each of the latter may contain an inclusion body. These giant cells are characteristic of chickenpox, zoster and herpes simplex virus infections (TZANCK and ARON-BRUNETIÈRE, 1949; BLANK *et al.*, 1951).

a) Histology of Skin Vesicles

The characteristic vesicular skin lesions in chickenpox have the same histopathological appearance as those in zoster, and this has been described by various authors (UNNA, 1896; TYZZER, 1905/06; LIPSCHÜTZ, 1921; DAHL, 1944). In vesicles of either clinical condition there is early involvement of the basal and deep prickle-cell layers of the epidermis. Intracellular and extracellular oedema develop, the former resulting in a "ballooning degeneration" of the affected cells, whilst the latter results in a separation of the prickle-cells so that a vesicle results with the roof formed by the outer cells of the prickle-cell layer as well as by the more external layers of the epidermis. The floor of the lesion may be formed by naked papillae of the corium or the remaining cells of the basal layer of the epidermis. The margins of the vesicle consist of cells undergoing "ballooning degeneration". In most cases a unilocular vesicle is formed, but multilocular vesicles do occur due to the rapid distension of a few liquefied cells (UNNA, 1896). The septa, however, are very thin and the vesicle usually collapses when pricked. The nuclear changes have been described above. Coincidental with the changes in the epidermis, perivascular infiltration of round cells occurs in the dermis, the endothelial cells of the lymph and blood vessels become swollen, and intranuclear inclusions develop in the latter cells in chickenpox (CHEATHAM et al., 1956). As the lesion evolves, polymorphonuclear leukocytes appear in increasing numbers in the corium and eventually predominate in the previously clear vesicle fluid, which also contains desquamated epithelial and "ballooned" cells. Healing of the vesicles eventually occurs by crusting, the crust becoming detached by the growth of subjacent epithelial cells.

b) Changes in Internal Organs

The incidence of chickenpox fatalities in a general population is not known but it is almost inconsequential (GORDON, 1962). Most of the autopsy reports are, therefore, on infants in the neonatal period where the mortality is 20 per cent (EHRLICH et al., 1958) or on adults with a complicated form of the disease. Probably the first description of specific pathological changes in the internal organs was by SCHLEUSSING in 1927 (quoted by EISENBUD, 1952) who reported areas of focal necrosis in the liver, adrenals and spleen in premature twins, three weeks old at the time of death. Inclusion bodies were not mentioned. Both OPPENHEIMER (1944) and LUCCHESI et al. (1947) who examined fatal neonatal cases, noted the striking affinity of the virus for epithelial cells in a wide variety of tissues, as judged by the occurrence of intranuclear inclusions. OPPENHEIMER regarded the virus as epidermotropic since there was an absence of inclusions in vascular endothelium. On the other hand, JOHNSON (1940) observed intranuclear inclusions, not only in the epithelial cells of the skin, oesophagus, renal pelvis, ureter and bile ducts, but also in endothelial cells of blood vessels and lymphatics, histiocytes, acinar cells of the pancreas, and medullary and cortical cells of the adrenal gland. In the case reported by CHEATHAM et al. (1956), intranuclear inclusions were found in capillary endothelial cells present in skin vesicles and in haemorrhagic areas in the testes, in vascular endothelium of the tongue and in endothelial cells in the thymus, lung, intestinal tract, liver, pancreas and kidneys. Autopsy observations on fatal cases of chickenpox associated with pneumonia (WARING et al., 1942; CLAUDY, 1947) revealed changes consistent with virus pneumonia, and both FRANK (1950) and EISENBUD (1952) described typical intranuclear inclusions in alveolar septal cells. In addition, KAPLAN and TULLY (1953) reported a patient with bronchogenic adenocarcinoma who had varicella inclusion bodies in both epithelial and mesenchymal tissues as well as in the adenocarcinoma cells of the lung.

The consistent histological findings in 6 cases of chickenpox encephalitis reviewed by APPELBAUM et al. (1953) were perivascular cellular infiltration and damage to the myelin similar to that found in the postinfectious encephalitides.

The widespread distribution of virus indicated by histopathological changes has been confirmed in the few virus studies that have been done on autopsy material. Thus, varicella virus has been isolated from the skin, blood, lungs and liver (CHEATHAM et al., 1956; EHRLICH et al., 1958; HAYES et al., 1965; WILLÉN et al., 1968).

4. Concurrent Infections

GORDON (1962) records the hospital experience of TOP (1941) for the period 1927—1936. During this time chickenpox and scarlet fever was the commonest combination of chickenpox and another communicable disease. Perhaps this is not so at the present time. GORDON (1962) also notes that chickenpox has been seen in combination with whooping cough, mumps, rubella and measles. CHRISTENSEN et al. (1953) noted the simultaneous occurrence of chickenpox and measles, and ARTENSTEIN and WEINSTEIN (1963) described the laboratory confirmation of concurrent chickenpox and measles in a patient and simultaneous infection with the two viruses in 4 of her 5 brothers. Both diseases took an apparently normal course but KNIGHT et al. (1964) reported a patient who had a "halo" area devoid of measles rash around chickenpox vesicles. The same phenomenon was noted by MERIGAN et al. (1968) in a patient whose chickenpox vesicles occurred before the measles rash. In other patients who developed measles and chickenpox concomitantly it seemed that the number of chickenpox vesicles was less than would otherwise have been expected.

B. Zoster

1. Clinical Aspects

The onset may be marked by malaise and fever which persist for 2 to 4 days, but there is usually pain from the beginning and often exquisite tenderness along the involved dorsal roots and their corresponding skin areas. These symptoms precede the appearance of the skin lesions by 1 to 12 days with, according to CARTER (1951), an average of 4 to 5 days. If the pain is severe, appendicitis, cholecystitis or pleurisy may be simulated (MOZHAEV, 1964; MALANINA, 1965) depending on the ganglia involved. In most patients pain disappears in 1 to 4 weeks. However, in 30 per cent of patients over 40 years, it persists as a post-zoster neuralgia for months or even years (BAMFORD and BOUNDY, 1968). It is most intractable in those who experience a long period of pre-herpetic symptoms and a severe eruption (HOPE-SIMPSON, 1967).

Nerve involvement without an eruption, otherwise known as "*zoster sine herpete*" may occur. LEWIS (1958) described 13 cases and suggested that zoster without any obvious skin eruption occurs more frequently than has been generally recognized.

The rash first appears at the point on the skin where the affected nerves come to the surface and spreads therefrom (STERN, 1937). It appears as groups of red macules which very rapidly vesiculate to form small, tense, clear vesicles on an erythematous base. During the next 7 days, and rarely longer, new groups of vesicles appear in fresh areas along the dermatome involved. After 5 to 10 days the vesicles have usually dried up to form scabs. Considerable scarring may occur (see p. 42). In addition, the regional lymph nodes are almost invariably enlarged and regress as the rash disappears (RAMOND and LEBEL, 1920).

One or more dermatomes may be involved but the disease is very rarely bilateral. It occurred in less than 0.5 per cent of 206 cases reported by BURGOON et al. (1957). The thoracic region is most commonly affected, the next being the areas of the neck and shoulders, supplied by the 2nd to 4th cervical ganglia, and the lumbar region (TAYLOR-ROBINSON, 1958; HOPE-SIMPSON, 1965). Of the cranial nerves, the ophthalmic division of the trigeminal is most frequently involved. 10 to 15 per cent of all zoster cases are of this sort (SEILER, 1949) and it has also been seen in a child (BIRKS, 1963). The eye itself is not affected in the majority of patients but some develop keratoconjunctivitis, which may appear with the skin lesions but more commonly follows them by 1 to 3 days. Residual scarring with impaired vision may ensue. Involvement of the geniculate ganglion results in vesicles in the external auditory meatus and facial paralysis. This association was first noted by KÖRNER (1904) but was described in more detail by HUNT (1907), whence it has been known as the Ramsay-Hunt syndrome (BRODY and WILKINS, 1968).

Generalized rash. TENNESON in 1893 (quoted by McEWEN, 1920) first used the term *"aberrant vesicles"* and the expressions *"herpes zoster generalisatus"*, *"herpes zoster varicellosus"* and *"disseminated herpes zoster"* found in the literature denote the generalized chickenpox-like eruption that occurs sometimes in zoster patients. The eruption has been described as appearing simultaneously with, and up to about one week after, the zoster rash (McEWEN, 1920; DAVIDSON, 1934; FERRIMAN, 1939; CAMPBELL, 1941; MERSELIS et al., 1964). SEILER (1949) estimated that 3.8 per cent of his zoster cases had an associated varicelliform rash and McCALLUM (1952) observed it in 7.6 per cent of his hospitalized zoster patients. BURGOON et al. (1957) recorded that 4 of 206 zoster patients (2 per cent), 55 years or older, had a generalized eruption. TAYLOR-ROBINSON (1958) observed a generalized rash in 12 (22 per cent) of 54 zoster patients, 6 of these rashes being profuse. Two children, $3\frac{1}{2}$ and 13 years old respectively, had a few "aberrant" vesicles only. Likewise, BOUGHTON (1966 b) noted an associated chickenpox-like rash in 23 per cent of his 123 hospitalized zoster patients. To what extent the element of selection of cases might affect the true incidence of a generalized rash is not possible to assess. Nor is it possible to assess whether others might have overlooked sparse vesicles. It seems likely, however, that sparse, widely distributed vesicles are not uncommon, and might be regarded as part of the normal zoster syndrome. Ulcers, similar to those in chickenpox, may be found on the buccal mucous membrane and result from vesicle rupture (BOUGHTON, 1966 b). The generalized rash itself resembles that of chickenpox but the characteristic polymorphism of the lesions in this condition is usually lacking and serves to differentiate between the two (HUTTON, 1935). The possible mechanism of occurrence is considered in the sections on Immunity and Pathogenesis (pp. 52 and 64).

2. Complications

a) Increased Severity

Zoster, like chickenpox, seems to occur more frequently in those with malignant disease, particularly lymphomas and lymphatic leukaemia. This was the clinical impression of CRAVER and HAAGENSEN (1932) and seems to have been substantiated since (RODNAN and RAKE, 1958; SHANBROM et al., 1960; WRIGHT and WINER, 1961; MILLER and BRUNELL, 1970). In addition, as judged by the greater duration of pain and frequency of a generalized rash it appears to be more severe in patients with malignant disease than in normal individuals (WILE and HOLMAN, 1940; DAYAN et al., 1964; MERSELIS et al., 1964; SOKAL and FIRAT, 1965; BRUNELL, 1968 personal communication). This is understandable, particularly in the reticuloses where production of circulating antibody may be defective, secondary hypogammaglobulinaemia may occur and where there may also be failure of cell-mediated immune mechanisms. BRUNELL et al. (1968) reported that zoster in children was similar to, but milder than, zoster in adults; one of their patients was being treated for leukaemia and another for Hodgkin's disease at the time zoster developed but the course of the latter was uneventful. KEIDAN and MAINWARING (1965) consider that the occurrence of zoster is more frequent in children with malignant disease, but, apart from haemorrhagic vesicles in two patients with profound thrombocytopenia, the zoster lesions they saw were neither severe nor extensive. Treatment of the underlying disease with corticosteroids, antimetabolites and alkylating agents did not appear to have an aggravating affect on the course of the zoster illness. RIFKIND (1966) saw uncomplicated disease in renal transplant patients who received immunosuppressive therapy. Such observations seem contrary to those of MULLER (1967) who considered zoster to be more severe in children with malignant disorders, and contrary to the observations of others who have observed severe zoster during the course of immunosuppressive therapy (BACON et al., 1965) and corticosteroid therapy (GOOD et al., 1957; ECKHARDT and HEBARD, 1961; FRY, 1963). To what extent such therapy aggravates zoster is, therefore, debatable since all the reports are based, no doubt necessarily, on subjective uncontrolled observations.

b) Central Nervous System Involvement

The central nervous system is probably involved to some extent in most cases since the cerebrospinal fluid regularly shows a lymphocytosis and an increase in globulin. Furthermore, varicella virus has been isolated from cerebrospinal fluid (GOLD and ROBBINS, 1958). Paralysis of motor nerves is well recognized (GRANT and ROWE, 1961; RUBIN and FUSFELD, 1965; BROSTOFF, 1966; GREENBERG, 1970) and is of the lower motor-neurone type and probably due to spread of virus to the anterior horn cells (HALPERN and COVNER, 1949). Meningoencephalitis or encephalitis has been described (SCHIFF and BRAIN, 1930; BRAIN, 1931; GORDON and TUCKER, 1945; KRUMHOLZ and LUHAN, 1945; APPELBAUM et al., 1962; HALL, 1963; PERIER et al., 1966).

3. Histopathological Changes

The histology of the skin vesicles in zoster is the same as in chickenpox and has been described previously (p. 38). However, in some cases of zoster the inflammatory reaction in the corium may be very severe, producing a destructive scarring lesion. Thus, in one case, 100 days after the onset, BROWDER and deVEER (1949) found scar tissue that could be traced from the surface of the skin deeply into the corium. In another case examined 34 months after the onset, small compact scars were situated chiefly within the dermis. They considered that the implication of nerve fibres in such scar tissue might explain the occurrence of post-herpetic neuralgia.

Changes in Central Nervous System

In addition to skin lesions, the virus in zoster produces a characteristic inflammatory reaction in the posterior nerve roots and ganglia. BRIGHT (1831) recognized that the segmental distribution of the zoster rash indicated nerve involvement and its neurological basis was supported by v. BÄRENSPRUNG (1862) who demonstrated a lesion in the posterior nerve-root ganglia corresponding to the cutaneous site of zoster. The classical work, however, is that of HEAD and CAMPBELL (1900) who made a detailed histological study of material from 21 persons who died between 3 and 790 days after the onset of the rash. They pointed out the uniform involvement of the spinal ganglia and other parts of the primary sensory neurone. In early lesions they observed haemorrhage and small round cell infiltration, both in the substance and in the sheath of the spinal ganglia, resulting in destruction of ganglion cells and fibres. The inflammatory changes extended into the dorsal nerve roots; after 13 days, degenerative changes, in the form of profound disintegration of the myelin nerve sheath, could be followed in the nerve fibres to the skin and in those passing centrally into, and for a variable distance along, the posterior columns of the spinal cord. A varying amount of secondary sclerosis occurred according to the severity of the acute destruction. The anterior root was normal in all cases.

The concept of zoster as a wider infection of the nervous system rather than a purely localized disease of the posterior root ganglia was put forward by LHERMITTE and his colleagues (quoted by GORDON and TUCKER, 1945). They showed that even in uncomplicated cases there are lesions not only of the posterior root ganglia but also of the anterior horns of those segments of the cord related to the affected ganglia. In addition, WOHLWILL (1924) drew attention to the posterior poliomyelitis present in cases of zoster, shown by a monocytic infiltration of the posterior horns and even of the bulb and cerebral peduncles. DENNY-BROWN et al. (1944) examined the spinal ganglia and other portions of the nervous system in 3 cases and drew attention to other changes apart from those in the spinal ganglia. They noted a unilateral myelitis, limited to 2 to 3 segments, involving chiefly the posterior horn and root with some changes in the anterior horn cells; a localized leptomeningitis limited to involved spinal segments and nerve roots; and finally, a true peripheral neuritis seen not only in the nerves distal to the ganglion but also in the anterior nerve root. Such lesions of the lower motor neurone, no doubt, account for those cases of muscular paralysis occurring in occasional cases of zoster.

The presence of inclusion bodies may be important evidence for the infection of nerve tissue by the virus. In no part of their work do HEAD and CAMPBELL (1900) mention such bodies. DENNY-BROWN et al. (1944) noted the absence of inclusions in the nerve tissues they examined, none of which was obtained earlier than the eleventh day after the onset of the disease. CHEATHAM (1953) first clearly described typical inclusion bodies in the affected nerve cells of a patient, with bilateral abdominal zoster and a generalized rash, who died on the eighth day of the zoster eruption. He found haemorrhage and necrosis in the dorsal root ganglia, with acidophilic intranuclear inclusions in both satellite and ganglion cells, those in the latter being larger and more basophilic than elsewhere. The sympathetic ganglion cells also occasionally contained intranuclear inclusion bodies. Again, CHEATHAM et al. (1956) described, in detail, the autopsy findings in a 4 year-old boy who presented a clinical picture of chickenpox but who was found to have, at postmortem, a typical zosteriform eruption along the tenth right dermatome in addition to disseminated chickenpox lesions. Dorsal root ganglia, T 6, T 9, T 10 and T 11 from the right side, were examined and inclusion bodies were found in the satellite cells of all; however, only rarely did ganglion cells in ganglia T 6 and

T 10 contain such inclusions. In one section of spinal cord, probably, it was said, from the lower thoracic region, there was minimal perivascular lymphocytic infiltration in the posterior columns and anterior horns but no inclusion bodies were seen, and no histological lesions of the brain were noted. In addition, in the zoster case mentioned above (CHEATHAM, 1953), inclusions were found in the myenteric plexus of the stomach, the oesophageal mucosa, the pancreas, ovary and adrenal gland as well as the skin itself. The inclusions were associated with areas of focal necrosis in the involved tissues.

McCORMICK et al. (1969) isolated varicella virus from the cerebrum of two cases of encephalomyelitis. ESIRI and TOMLINSON (1972) did not isolate virus but presented electron microscope evidence for its presence in the skin, the first division of the trigeminal nerve and ganglion of a woman who died four days after the onset of ophthalmic zoster. Virus particles were found in nuclei and cytoplasm of epidermal cells of the skin. The frontal nerve showed degenerate axons and myelin in some bundles and viral antigen was detected by immunofluorescence in 2 of 11 bundles; virus particles were seen in the cytoplasm of perineurial cells and in both cytoplasm and nuclei of Schwann cells. Viral antigen was demonstrated in one bundle of the ophthalmic nerve. In some areas of the trigeminal ganglion there was ganglion cell degeneration and disarray of satellite cells; in both types of cells there were virus particles in the nucleus and cytoplasm. The findings suggest that varicella virus spreads in peripheral nerves by growth in endoneural cells rather than by transport in a "conduit" as seems to be the case with rabies virus.

In conclusion, therefore, it may be seen that the histopathological changes in chickenpox and zoster are essentially the same. Zoster is an infection generally limited to the central nervous system, but generalization of the virus results in identical histopathological changes in the same diverse tissues as seen in fatal cases of chickenpox. It would seem that in both chickenpox and zoster with a generalized rash, the virus is carried to the tissues via the blood stream; it would be difficult to conceive of any other mechanism to account for the wide range of tissues involved and the finding of intranuclear inclusions in vascular endothelial cells supports this idea. Basically, the vesicles of the two diseases are identical. The presence of intranuclear inclusions in vascular endothelium in relation to chickenpox vesicles and the failure, up to the present time, to demonstrate such endothelial inclusions in relation to vesicles of the uncomplicated zoster rash is interesting and points, possibly, to a purely nerve transportation of virus to the skin in uncomplicated zoster. The claim for marked dermotropism and neutrotropism of the virus in chickenpox and zoster, respectively, is not supported by careful histopathological examination of fatal cases, in which epithelial and endothelial cells have been found to be involved in both diseases.

C. Considerations of the Association of Varicella Virus with Other Clinical Entities

1. Foetal Malformation

Chromosomal aberrations have been reported to occur in varicella virus infections. AULA (1963) looked at manually squashed chromosomes and reported an increase in breaks during the first days of chickenpox. This technique may lead to false conclusions but similar results were obtained by AULA (1964) when the chromosome spread was made by air drying. GRIPENBERG (1965) found an increased number of breaks in chromosomes of leukocytes from 1 of 3 cases of chickenpox. MASSIMO et al. (1965) reported the occurrence of chickenpox in a mother during the sixth month of pregnancy, the baby having premature closing of the fontanelles, microcephaly, micrognathia and a large number of chromosome breaks; the technique of chromosome spread was not mentioned. Such reports seem consistent with the ability of varicella virus to produce chromosomal changes in tissue-culture cells (p. 26), but it is not possible to judge the true situation on a single case or on studies which are ill-controlled. In this respect, the study of CHUN et al. (1966) is relevant. They examined leukocytes from 10 children in the early days of chickenpox illness and from 12 healthy children. Some chromosomal abnormalities were seen but they were no more frequent in the chickenpox group than in the control group. HARNDEN (1964) also found no excess of abnormalities in leukocyte chromosomes from 7 cases of zoster or from 5 cases of chickenpox, and neither did GROUCHY et al. (1967) in 3 cases of chickenpox.

Whether or not varicella virus produces chromosomal abnormalities in natural infections, there is practically no reliable evidence that it causes foetal malformations (FISH, 1965; HARDY, 1965), although infection may take place in utero (p. 53). Multiple congenital defects in the baby of a mother who had chickenpox in the eighth week of pregnancy have been described (LAFORET and LYNCH, 1947) but several comprehensive studies (SWAN and TOSTEVIN, 1946; SWAN et al., 1946; FOX et al., 1948; HILL et al., 1958; DUMONT, 1960) have not revealed proof that chickenpox is a cause of foetal abnormalities or that it is a significant cause of foetal death (SIEGEL et al., 1966), or that it leads to prematurity or low birth weight (MANSON et al., 1960; SIEGEL and FUERST, 1966). In the light of these findings, the reports by DUEHR (1955) and others of anomalies in infants born of mothers who had zoster in pregnancy are not suggestive of a direct causal association.

2. Multiple Sclerosis

ROSS et al. (1965 a) examined single sera from 96 cases of multiple sclerosis and from 96 matched controls for complement-fixing antibodies to a variety of infectious agents including varicella virus. Antibody for each of the agents was present in a greater number of patients than controls but a statistically significant difference was obtained only with varicella virus. Several reasons for the finding were proposed: that patients with multiple sclerosis might react differently to infectious agents than normal persons; that they might be particularly susceptible to infection with varicella virus; that infection with varicella virus might be associated with the aetiology of multiple sclerosis. If the latter were the case, these workers considered that the virus might remain latent in the central nervous system and that its reactivation might be associated with clinical relapse and a rise in antibody titre. They collected serial sera from 13 patients who had clinical relapses and also from 17 patients with retrobulbar neuritis but failed to detect rises in complement-fixing antibody to varicella virus or measles or herpes simplex viruses (ROSS et al., 1969). Thus, there was no support for the idea that virus reactivation might give rise to an acute exacerbation of the disease. On the other hand, the continued high titre of antibody detected in 2 patients with multiple sclerosis might be a cumulative effect of periodic reactivation. Clearly, however, any causative association between varicella virus and multiple sclerosis is at the moment in doubt.

3. Facial Palsy

AITKEN and BRAIN (1933) studied the association between varicella virus and facial palsy be means of the complement-fixation test in which they used fluid from zoster vesicles as antigen. They found that sera from all 9 patients suffering from the Ramsay-Hunt syndrome fixed complement whereas only 4 of those from 22 patients with Bell's palsy without a zoster eruption did so. DODGE and POSKANZER (1962) could not detect a rise in complement-fixing antibody to varicella virus in sera from 4 patients with Bell's palsy, nor did they find a rise in complement-fixing antibody to herpes simplex virus in the sera of 5 other persons with this disease. Because of the availability of potent complement-fixing antigens of varicella virus, PEITERSEN and CAUNT (1970) examined a further series of 27 Bell's palsy cases serologically to see whether any could be shown to be 'zoster sine herpete'. Sera from 5 patients only reacted with a zoster complement-fixing antigen and four of these had typical zoster eruptions. Thus only 1 case of 'zoster sine herpete' was found, and for the most part the aetiology of Bell's palsy remains unknown.

VIII. Immunity

As indicated previously (p. 34) man is probably the only species susceptible to varicella virus. Evidence for infection of other primates is minimal and other laboratory animals exhibit complete resistance to growth of the virus.

A. Experimental Human Infections

Successful transfer of varicella virus was first performed by STEINER (1875) who was able to reproduce chickenpox eruptions by inoculating children with the contents of chickenpox vesicles. KLING (1915) observed that following cutaneous inoculation of fresh chickenpox vesicle fluid, some children failed to react, others developed local vesicles at the site of inoculation and in a few a generalized rash followed a few days later. On the other hand, HESS and UNGAR (1918) and GULÁCSY (1933) inoculated children without success. However, they do not comment on the appearance or age of their fluids so that their failure could have been due to lack of infectious virus in the material which they inoculated.

KUNDRATITZ (1925) carried out similar experiments with fluid from zoster vesicles and was able to produce a chickenpox-like rash in 2 of 28 children he inoculated cutaneously. BRUUSGAARD (1932) observed chickenpox rashes in 4 of 18 children he inoculated with zoster vesicle fluid. Whether the rashes were of true chickenpox distribution is impossible to know but that they were due to virus is suggested by the fact that KUNDRATITZ failed to infect with chickenpox vesicle fluid those children who had recovered from infection induced by fluid from zoster vesicles and likewise, inoculation of fluid from vesicles had no effect in children who had had chickenpox. The experimental inoculation of adults with chickenpox vesicle material failed to produce lesions in any, confirming the presence of immunity in the group as contrasted with young children (BRUUSGAARD, 1932).

B. Second Attacks of Natural Infections

1. Chickenpox

Recovery from chickenpox is usually associated with a solid immunity to reinfection. The Medical Research Council School Epidemic Committee (1938) was of the opinion that the number of reputed second attacks was not more than might easily be accounted for by errors in medical histories. It is generally agreed, however, that second attacks do occur. MITCHELL and FLETCHER (1927) obtained a history of previous chickenpox infection in 9 out of 775 chickenpox cases. Of course, as indicated above, a history provided by the patient is unreliable (KASS et al., 1952) and it seems unlikely that the secondary attack rate is as high as 1 per cent. In addition, other authors (HUGHES and SMITH, 1939; CRISP, 1940; GRIVEL, 1941) have recorded instances of second attacks. In 1940, a medical practitioner reported that his 13 year-old son had had 4 attacks (LEAK, 1940). Clearly, such an occurrence is a rarity and it is not known whether there was a contributory factor such as agammaglobulinaemia.

2. Zoster

It is a misconception that an attack of zoster results in life-long immunity. Second attacks have been recorded (HEAD and CAMPBELL, 1900), with lesions on the opposite side (GRAHAM-LITTLE, 1937) and on the same side of the body as the original zoster eruption (SEILER, 1949). The latter author found recurrent zoster in 3.3 per cent of his cases and, apart from one case, a period of 20 years or more elapsed between the two occurrences. KASS et al. (1952) obtained a history of previous zoster in 3 (4.2 per cent) of their 72 patients. The series of 192 zoster cases observed by HOPE-SIMPSON (1965) comprised 8 (4.2 per cent) which were recorded as second attacks and one as a third attack. Multiple occurrence had been observed previously (Medical Research Council School Epidemic Committee, 1938) and might be associated with immunosuppressive or cytotoxic drug therapy (Brit. med. J., 1968). HOPE-SIMPSON considered that the high secondary attack rate he noted might be an under-estimate because enquiry regarding second attacks of zoster was not specifically made in the earlier years of his study. Nevertheless, the incidence of zoster among those who had already had an attack was at least as high as that of first attacks in the general population. On the evidence there seems little reasons to suspect the relatively high frequency of second zoster attacks. It is worth noting, however, that several cases originally diagnosed as recurrent zoster by BLANK and RAKE (1955) were all found to have recurrent zosteriform herpes simplex infections by serological and virus isolation studies.

C. Serological Investigations

Serological studies in the last decade have been concerned not only with the relationship between the viruses isolated from chickenpox and zoster patients (p. 13) but also with the immune response of the patient, the persistence and placental transfer of antibody and the relationship of antibody to immunity.

1. Development of Antibody in Chickenpox and Zoster Infections

a) Complement-Fixation Tests

WELLER and WITTON (1958) reported a more rapid rise in complement-fixing antibody titre in zoster than in chickenpox cases although by the convalescent stage of the illnesses the level of antibody was the same in each condition. TAYLOR-ROBINSON and DOWNIE (1959) confirmed the more rapid rise of antibody in zoster but in their patients it reached a higher titre in zoster than in chickenpox. The same observation was made by MILLER and BRUNELL (1970). Ross et al. (1965 b) and CAUNT and SHAW (1969) have noted high titres of complement-fixing antibody in some sera taken in the first 10 days of chickenpox illnesses, and this was probably due to the use of more potent antigens than those used by previous investigators.

b) Gel-Diffusion Tests

Quantitative differences in the antibody response of chickenpox and zoster patients were observed in precipitation tests using the Ouchterlony technique (TAYLOR-ROBINSON and RONDLE, 1959). All convalescent-phase sera from zoster patients, taken 3 to 4 weeks after the onset of the eruption, produced precipitation lines with fluids from zoster and chickenpox vesicles; half of the sera collected in the first week after the eruption produced positive reactions also. On the other hand, acute or convalescent-phase sera from chickenpox patients failed to produce precipitation and convalescent-phase sera only did so when they were concentrated five-fold. The results indicated an earlier and greater antibody response in patients with zoster than in those with chickenpox. In contrast, TRLIFAJOVÁ et al. (1970) found that precipitating antibody occurred in the sera of chickenpox patients as early in their illnesses as it did in zoster patients. This they attributed to the use of a potent antigen, but other details of their technique (see p. 16) also differed from that of TAYLOR-ROBINSON and RONDLE (1959). These factors may also account for the greater proportion of positive precipitation tests detected by TRLIFAJOVÁ et al. (1970), i.e. in 7 of 10 chickenpox cases in the first week of illness.

c) Neutralization Tests

WELLER and WITTON (1958) found that undiluted sera from early cases of chickenpox did not have neutralizing activity as frequently as comparable sera from cases of zoster, and in titration of two convalescent-phase sera, serum from a case of chickenpox had a lower antibody titre than serum from a case of zoster. TAYLOR-ROBINSON (1959) obtained similar results but dilutions of sera were not tested so that, although it was shown that complete neutralization of varicella virus was affected by convalescent-phase sera from both chickenpox and zoster patients, it was not possible to demonstrate that convalescent-phase zoster sera had higher titres of neutralizing antibody than comparable chickenpox sera. CAUNT and SHAW (1969) did quantitative neutralization tests and found that the antibody response of chickenpox patients was poor, the maximum titre demonstrated being 1 : 40. Early acute-phase sera from zoster patients had very low titres of neutralizing antibody or undetectable amounts but high titres of antibody developed rapidly in the sera of these patients.

It is clear that the results of all the serological tests, in particular the earlier and greater antibody response observed in cases of zoster as opposed to cases of chickenpox, support the view that zoster is a second clinical manifestation of infection by varicella virus.

2. Persistence of Antibody

a) After Chickenpox

Complement-fixation tests on serial sera obtained over various periods of time have been done by a few workers. WELLER (1957) detected antibody in sera from chickenpox patients 1 to 4 years after the eruption. TAYLOR-ROBINSON and DOWNIE (1959) reported that complement-fixing antibody was not usually detectable in sera taken some 6 months or more after a clinical attack of chickenpox. GOLD and GODEK (1965) tested 103 sera from 72 persons with chickenpox. Elevated levels of complement-fixing antibody were detected for 3 months after the rash but then there was a gradual decline so that less than 25 per cent of persons had detectable antibody in their sera 1 year later. Differences in results may reflect differences in the sensitivity of the tests used by each worker but it seems clear that complement-fixing antibody wanes within a few months of an attack of chickenpox.

Even less data are available concerning the persistence of neutralizing antibody after an attack of chickenpox. It wanes gradually and persists longer than complement-fixing antibody. Thus, five sera collected between 13 and 40 years after the initial illness contained some neutralizing antibody but no complement-fixing antibody (TAYLOR-ROBINSON, 1959). These sera were tested undiluted and quantitative estimations of antibody content were not made. However, CAUNT and SHAW (1969) used a quantitative technique to test sera from nine adults who had chickenpox 20 to 40 years previously. Six of these had neutralizing antibody titres of 1 : 10 or less which would be consistent with a gradual decline from an original low level. Certainly, those who develop zoster in later life do not have detectable amounts of neutralizing antibody to varicella virus when this illness occurs (CAUNT and SHAW, 1969), so that antibody must have waned in such subjects. The sera of one person tested by CAUNT and SHAW 20 and 30 years after chickenpox contained high levels of neutralizing antibody. This might have been due to reversion of latent varicella virus to virus capable of stimulating antibody, as postulated by HOPE-SIMPSON (1965), or to subclinical re-infection with varicella virus. While GOLD and GODEK (1965) could not produce evidence to support the latter possibility, CAUNT and SHAW (1969) did think it was feasible. They observed a rise in the titre of neutralizing antibody in the sera of a mother who did not develop chickenpox but whose children had done so.

b) After Zoster

WELLER (1957) reported the presence of complement-fixing antibody 1 to 4 years after both zoster and chickenpox. On the other hand, TAYLOR-ROBINSON (1958) although not examining many serial sera, thought that complement-fixing antibody declined rapidly after zoster. He could not detect complement-fixing antibody in the sera of two zoster patients, taken 107 and 120 days respectively from the onset of the rash. GOLD and GODEK (1965) were of the same opinion. They examined 51 sera from 21 cases of zoster and reported that the fall in complement-fixing antibody titre proceeded similarly to that after chickenpox. RIFKIND (1966) noted that a complement-fixing antibody titre of 1 : 256 detected 30 days after the onset of zoster had 5½ months later fallen to 1 : 16.

CAUNT and SHAW (1969) examined sera from 5 persons who had had zoster one month to 40 years previously. All had high levels of neutralizing antibody although sera from one patient showed at least a four-fold fall in titre after two years. These results clearly suggest that neutralizing antibody persists longer than complement-fixing antibody after zoster, but there is insufficient evidence to be certain whether neutralizing antibody persists for a longer period after zoster than after chickenpox. Sera from persons who have suffered multiple attacks of zoster have not been examined to determine whether neutralizing antibody is at a low level at the time of the second or third attack.

c) In the Sera of Persons in Different Age Groups

Little information is available concerning the varicella virus antibody status of healthy persons of different ages in the general population. Recently, TOMLINSON and MacCALLUM (1970) examined by the complement-fixation technique 184 sera sent to their Oxford laboratory between January and August 1967 and 183 sera from blood donors. The lowest proportion of sera with detectable antibody was in the age group 0—10 years. Thereafter the proportion of sera within each 10 years age group containing detectable antibody was over 70 per cent with a gradual decline with increasing age most noticeable in the sera of blood donors in the age group 41—60 years. After the age of 70 years there was an increase in the proportion of sera that contained detectable antibody. These workers point out that the apparent decrease in incidence of complement-fixing antibody to varicella virus with advancing years is in contrast to the gradual increase in antibody to herpes simplex virus reported by SMITH et al. (1967). A few sera from persons of different ages were tested also by SCHMIDT et al. (1969) who used the complement-fixation technique. Their results suggested that sera from persons older than 31 years of age contained antibody less frequently than sera from persons 11 to 30 years. Such results are indicative of a decline in complement-fixing antibody following chickenpox but, of course, the picture is complex because re-exposure to chickenpox and zoster must have occurred in some of the individuals.

3. Antibody and Its Relationship to Immunity

a) Antibody Class

BRUNELL (1966) used sucrose density centrifugation to show that the complement-fixing antibody which developed in chickenpox infections was mainly IgG and that in some cases there was placental transfer (p. 51). RIFKIND (1966) used gel filtration to show that the antibody in serum obtained from a zoster patient 17 days after the onset of the rash had IgG characteristics. It is, however, difficult to reconcile this with his finding that 2-mercaptoethanol treatment of several sera from zoster patients destroyed their content of complement-fixing antibody. SHAW (1968), by the same treatment, was not able to destroy complement-fixing or neutralizing activity in the sera of 3 convalescent zoster patients which suggests the presence of IgG antibody. He did not, however, include in his tests a serum which contained antibody known to be destroyed by 2-mercaptoethanol. However, the results of the filtration and centrifugation studies clearly indicate the development of IgG antibody.

LEONARD et al. (1970) separated the various classes of γ-globulins by DEAE-cellulose chromatography and found IgM antibodies with varicella virus neutralizing activity in chickenpox convalescent-phase sera, but not in zoster convalescent-phase sera. They found two subclasses of IgG, one of which migrated more rapidly than the other. Virus neutralizing activity was present in both subclasses of convalescent-phase zoster sera but only in the slow moving fraction of chickenpox convalescent-phase sera. These authors suggest that most protective ability resides in the fast moving IgG fraction of the neutralizing antibody and that the antibody response in chickenpox is incomplete.

Further observations on the relationship of antibody to immunity are based on the type of serological test that has been used to measure antibody.

b) Complement-Fixing Antibody

It may seem irrelevant to consider antibody measured by the complement-fixation technique in relation to immunity because that measured by the neutralization technique is clearly more important. However, a positive result in a complement-fixation test is an indication that neutralizing antibody is present also and there is some evidence to indicate that the presence of complement-fixing antibody in the serum of a newborn infant may be correlated with immunity. Laboratory studies on the placental transfer of antibody directed against varicella virus had not received attention until recently. BRUNELL (1966) found that if more than 5 days elapsed between the onset of maternal chickenpox or zoster and delivery the serum complement-fixing antibody titre of the newborn was similar to that of the mother, whose antibody was predominantly IgG. If the interval was shorter, the titre of complement-fixing antibody in cord serum was lower than in the mother's serum or was not detectable at all, possibly due to insufficient time for placental transfer of antibody. Four of 5 mothers who developed chickenpox within a week before delivery gave birth to live infants, one of which developed chickenpox. This infant had no complement-fixing antibody in the cord serum while the 3 other infants did, suggesting that the presence of antibody detectable by the complement-fixation technique might prevent neonatal infection (BRUNELL, 1967 a).

On the other hand, the absence of complement-fixing antibody is not an indication of lack of immunity and there is ample evidence for this. GOLD and GODEK (1965) noted that a fall in complement-fixing antibody titre to an undetectable level following chickenpox or zoster was not accompanied by any apparent change in susceptibility to varicella virus. Immunity persisted, second attacks of chickenpox or zoster not being seen, presumably due to the persistence of neutralizing antibody. These authors considered that the complement-fixation technique was of little value in determining susceptibility to infection. RIFKIND (1966) reported that complement-fixing antibody to varicella virus did not develop in two patients who developed zoster during the course of lymphatic leukaemia and that a generalized rash occurred in each. On the contrary, GOLD (1966) observed a patient with chronic lymphatic leukaemia in whom complement-fixing antibody did not develop during the first 18 days of a zoster illness and yet this was not severe, while other persons who rapidly developed complement-fixing antibody suffered severe zoster illnesses. Gold suggested that the level of complement-fixing antibody did not determine the severity of the illness, a point also brought out by MILLER and BRUNELL (1970).

c) Neutralizing Antibody

READETT and McGIBBON (1961) observed chickenpox in 2 infants 12 to 14 days after birth, the infections having been contracted from members of the families other than the mothers. Neutralizing antibody was shown to be present in the mothers' sera but the cord sera were not examined. The infrequency of cases such as this when opportunities for their occurrence are so frequent indicates that usually there is placental transfer of protective antibody which, although there are no data for its support, must surely be neutralizing antibody. It seems that chickenpox in children occurs when this passively transferred antibody has disappeared. In keeping with this is the fact that persons who develop chickenpox, or indeed zoster, invariably lack neutralizing antibody at the onset of the rash (TAYLOR-ROBINSON, 1959; CAUNT and SHAW, 1969). This finding is not at variance with the view of HOPE-SIMPSON (1965) that zoster occurs in those whose immunity has fallen to a negligible level due to the varicella virus being sequestered in a latent form away from the antibody-forming system and so not providing a continuous antigenic stimulus. This concept and the possible reason for such persons developing zoster and not a second attack of chickenpox are considered further (pp. 63 and 64). The mechanism whereby a generalized varicelliform rash occurs during the course of some cases of zoster is unknown but lack of vesicular interferon production (ARMSTRONG et al., 1970) may be an important factor. The speed of neutralizing antibody production in such cases is unknown but it is interesting that STEVENS and MERIGAN (1971) find the development of complement-fixing antibody delayed in disseminated zoster.

4. Passive Immunization with γ-Globulin

There are conflicting reports regarding passive immunity conferred by the inoculation of human γ-globulin and these are discussed in relation to prophylactic immunization (p. 65). CAUNT and SHAW (1969) pointed out that many adults have very low levels of neutralizing antibody to varicella virus in their sera and that it would not be surprising to find that some batches of γ-globulin produced from pooled sera were ineffective. Convalescent-phase zoster sera have the highest titres of neutralizing antibody and, in addition, they contain a type of antibody not seen in convalescent-phase chickenpox sera and which may have particular neutralizing capacity (LEONARD et al., 1970). It would, therefore, be wise to use such zoster sera in prophylaxis, as done by ABRAMSON (1944), or to use γ-globulin prepared from them (BRUNELL et al., 1969).

IX. Epidemiology

A. Sex Incidence

The incidence of chickenpox in males and females is about equal. GORDON (1962) noted that of 159,512 cases of chickenpox that were reported in Massachusetts during the years 1952—1961, 52 per cent were males and 48 per cent females.

In contrast, there is some controversy about the sex incidence of zoster. DAHL (1946) found that of 798 hospitalized cases of zoster in Copenhagen over a 5-year period, 484 were in males and 314 in females. Similarly, HELLGREN and HERSLE (1966) saw a preponderance of male zoster patients coming to a hospital in Gothenburg. SEILER (1949) thought that the preponderance of male cases that he saw might be due to the larger number of men attending for hospital treatment. On the other hand, McGREGOR (1957) and BURGOON et al. (1957) noted no significant difference in incidence by sex. The latter workers noted that of their 206 patients 50.7 per cent were males and 49.3 per cent females as compared with the total Philadelphia population of 48.3 per cent male and 51.7 per cent female. HOPE-SIMPSON (1965) also could not support the idea that males suffered from zoster more frequently than females and was sceptical about figures drawn from hospital experience because of the uncertain manner of selection of the patients.

B. Age Incidence

1. Chickenpox

a) Congenital

If the rash is present at birth or occurs within 10 days of birth, then it seems that there must have been transplacental passage of varicella virus. HUBBARD (1878) was the first to report such a case, the rash occurring 24 hours after birth. GORDON (1962) gathered from the literature 24 instances of chickenpox in newborn infants all occurring within 10 days of birth; 16 mothers gave a history of chickenpox within the final days of pregnancy, varying from 10 days to one day before birth. However, obtaining a history of chickenpox or observing it in the mother is not always possible and, indeed, there is evidence for inapparent infection in the mother (PRIDHAM, 1913). PEARSON (1964) observed that 16 mothers had chickenpox at the time of delivery but it occurred in only 6 of their infants soon after birth. As pointed out by HYATT (1967) in a review of 34 cases of chickenpox which occurred in the first 10 days of life, mothers with chickenpox more often than not give birth to infants without the disease. Adequate time for the development of maternal antibody and for its transplacental passage is probably a factor influencing the occurrence of chickenpox in the newborn (see p. 51).

b) Neonatal

This is regarded as chickenpox acquired by contact soon after birth. Two clear instances are reported by READETT and McGIBBON (1961). In both cases the mother did not have chickenpox, the disease in the infant being contracted from a member of the family. GORDON (1962) collected 8 other cases from the literature in which chickenpox occurred 11 to 20 days after delivery. However, there was no clear evidence of whether infection was of congenital or postnatal origin.

c) In Children and Adults

The disease occurs for the most part in children under 10 years of age with greatest prevalence between 3 and 6 years (RIVERS and ELDRIDGE, 1929). This is substantiated by the finding that 90 per cent of the reported cases in Massachusetts during the years 1952—1961 were in children before the age of 10 years and the maximum observed incidence by years of life was at the age of 6 years (GORDON, 1962). In Sweden, in contrast to the decline in whooping cough, scarlet fever and measles, the incidence of chickenpox in children born in 1949 was the same as for those born in 1939, but the onset was seen less frequently in those aged 8—12 years and more frequently in those aged 0—4 years (STRÖM, 1967). According to the Medical Research Council Special Report (1938) about 67 per cent of boys and 60 per cent of girls had had chickenpox before secondary school entry, that is before 11 to 12 years of age. Chickenpox in a 76 year-old woman (ROLLESTON, 1932) and in an 85 year-old (ROTEM, 1961) has been observed, and in a tropical climate chickenpox has been observed to occur more frequently in older age groups (MARETIĆ and COORAY, 1963). Furthermore, it may occur more particularly in adults who have not previously been exposed to varicella virus (BARNETT, 1950).

2. Zoster

a) In the Newborn

The occurrence of zoster in the newborn has been reported by several authors (LOMER, 1889; KALB, 1909; TAUSCH, 1932; BONAR and PEARSALL, 1932; FREUD et al., 1942; COUNTER and KORN, 1950; FELDMAN, 1952; ADKISSON, 1965) but despite this it is rare. KATAYAMA (1938) noted zoster in the newborn only once in a series of 487 cases of zoster. Some of the reports certainly seem to be clinically convincing. However, apart from FELDMAN (1952) who made an effort to show that the virus was not herpes simplex, none of the reports is supported by laboratory evidence of varicella virus infection.

b) In Children and Adults

As opposed to its occurrence in the newborn, zoster in young children is undoubted (TAYLOR-ROBINSON, 1958; WINKELMANN and PERRY, 1959; BRUNELL et al., 1968). However, in contrast to chickenpox, zoster most frequently appears in the later decades of life. DAHL (1946) found that less than 5 per cent of his cases were under 10 years of age. Sixty per cent of patients seen by SEILER (1949) were over 45 years of age, almost half of those seen by KASS et al. (1952) were between 50 and 69 years of age, and 60 per cent of the zoster cases seen by TAYLOR-ROBINSON (1958) were between 50 and 80 years of age. Further, HOPE-SIMPSON (1965) found that the rate of occurrence increased in the older age groups and was particularly marked in those aged 50 years and more.

C. Seasonal Incidence

Chickenpox is essentially an epidemic disease and has a seasonal variation with a prevalence in the winter and spring (GORDON, 1962). In a tropical climate, as for example in Ceylon, there is seasonal variation also, more cases being seen in the dry than in the monsoon season (MARETIĆ and COORAY, 1963).

Zoster has been considered by some to have a seasonal occurrence. v. Bókay (1928) reported that he encountered it more frequently in June and the autumn months. Head and Campbell (1900) while recognizing the sporadic incidence, also noted from the London Hospital records an increase in the number of cases seen at certain times of the year. Likewise, Hellgren and Hersle (1966) recorded a higher incidence of cases in June, July and August, a finding apparently consistent from year to year in patients in hospital and attending hospital clinics. However, the assessment of incidence on the basis of those cases admitted to hospital is difficult and the results of several other studies seem to indicate that there is no marked seasonal variation in the incidence of zoster. When the mean of a large number of cases over a period of many years was plotted, the curve indicating the monthly incidence of zoster approached a straight line (Rivers and Eldridge, 1929). Kass et al. (1952), and Burgoon et al. (1957) in an analysis of their 206 cases, found no statistically valid difference in the incidence of zoster in any of the four seasons. Furthermore, both McGregor (1957) and Hope-Simpson (1965) from studies of patients at home came to the conclusion that the occurrence of zoster was independent of any seasonal influence.

D. The Occurence of Disease in Contacts of Chickenpox and Zoster

1. Chickenpox after Contact with Chickenpox

a) Endemicity and Epidemicity

Chickenpox has been observed in practically every part of the world (Simons et al., 1944). The pattern is usually a fluctuating endemic one with epidemics recurring every few years. Gordon (1962) commented upon the behaviour of chickenpox in the state of Massachusetts over a period of 50 years from 1910. Epidemic peaks were noted every 2 to 4 years. A similar epidemic periodicity was recorded by Hope-Simpson (1965) in a rural area of England.

b) Communicability

Chickenpox is communicable from person to person and this is the usual mode of spread although a chickenpox epidemic may be initiated by a case of zoster. Usually just less than three-fourths of susceptible contacts of chickenpox develop the disease, a figure derived from observations of outbreaks in hospital wards (Gordon and Meader, 1929; Gordon, 1962). In affected households 61 per cent of susceptible children aged 0 to 15 years contract chickenpox, but only 12 per cent of apparent susceptibles above that age (Simpson, 1952; 1954). The lower rate among older persons is probably due to previous inapparent infections and an inability to recall past events. The attack rate for measles is higher than for chickenpox but it is lower for rubella and for mumps.

2. Chickenpox after Contact with Zoster

a) Evidence for the Association

Although chickenpox usually spreads from case to case, the occurrence of chickenpox in contacts of zoster is undoubted. v. Bókay (1909) first drew attention to this and continued to do so in later publications (1919, 1924, 1928). Since then many instances of this particular relationship have been recorded (Cowie, 1925; Netter, 1928; Blatt et al., 1940; Garland, 1943; Peterson and Black, 1946; Seiler, 1949; Simpson, 1954; Brodkin, 1963; Hope-Simpson, 1965; Weingarten, 1965). The Medical Research Council School Epidemic Committee (1938) reported that during the period of 5 years from 1930—1934, 20 outbreaks of chickenpox were preceded by a zoster case, and in 18 of these outbreaks the date of onset of the first case of chickenpox was such that the preceding zoster might have been the infecting agent. Pickles (1939) stated that on more than one occasion the association had been taken for granted by his patients who could not have acquired the knowledge from medical books, and Le Feuvre (1917) concludes in his paper: "A thing that one may so often confidently expect can surely scarcely be called a coincidence."

b) Communicability

Seiler (1949) estimated that the chickenpox attack rate in susceptibles exposed to zoster cases was 15 per cent. It is clear, therefore, that chickenpox occurs less frequently from exposure to a case of zoster than it does from exposure to a case of chickenpox (Gordon, 1962). There would seem to be two reasons for this. Firstly, the lesions in zoster are often covered and there is rarely involvement of respiratory tract mucosa. Secondly, because zoster occurs mainly in older persons their contacts are more likely to be immune adults rather than susceptible children.

3. Zoster after Contact with Chickenpox or Zoster

a) Evidence for the Association

v. Bókay (quoted by Le Feuvre, 1917) remarked on the absence up to 1909 of any evidence of chickenpox being followed by zoster, but added "it is quite probable that once attention has been drawn to the aetiological connection between the two diseases, one will have opportunities of observing this reverse sequence". In 1924 v. Bókay, in appraising both his own observations and those of others, concluded that chickenpox gave rise to zoster in contacts one-seventh as commonly as the reverse. However, his attempts (1924 and 1928) to draw a parallel between the incidence of chickenpox and zoster in Budapest, between 1915 and 1924 are not convincing. Netter (1928) collected 174 examples of chickenpox following zoster and 25 cases of the reverse in which he considered the incubation period was the same. Furthermore, the Medical Research Council School Epidemic Committee (1938) reported that there were 8 instances over a 5-year period in which a case of chickenpox was followed by cases of zoster and in only one instance did it seem unlikely to them that the initial case of chickenpox was the source of infection for the associated zoster. Since then Horton (1948), Moscovitz (1955), and Reich and Baumal (1961) have also commented upon the occurrence of zoster in persons coming in contact with chickenpox. Of course, this association is more likely to be seen in children who develop zoster (Golemba, 1958) than in adults.

Zoster is usually a sporadic disease and evidence supporting the idea that zoster gives rise to zoster in exposed individuals is scant. Fuhlrott (1920) reported 10 cases occurring "within a few days" in a prisoner-of-war camp of

1,400 men, and LEVADITI (1926) referred to a number of small "epidemics" and mentioned the work of BALDET who wrote a thesis (1895) on zoster epidemics. Most recently, RADO et al. (1965) described a small epidemic of zoster occurring in a hospital ward, although it is not absolutely clear whether or not some of the cases might have been chickenpox. BARNETT (1950) and HOPE-SIMPSON (1965) also have observed zoster to occur in a person after contact with zoster about 2 to 3 weeks previously. However, HOPE-SIMPSON considers that if the association is a real one it is a very rare event indeed.

b) Evidence against the Association

SEILER (1949) found that a history of recent contact with chickenpox before zoster was given by 14 of 184 patients (in 8 through a third party only) and in only 3 of the remaining 6 cases were the circumstances really suggestive of association. Other common infections occurred in approximately the same proportion which suggests that the chickenpox association might well have been fortuitous.

Attempts to obtain from patients with zoster a history of recent contact with chickenpox or with other cases of zoster usually provide equivocal answers (TAYLOR-ROBINSON, 1958). However, TAYLOR-ROBINSON (1958) could not find evidence of zoster developing in members of 28 families in which one or more cases of chickenpox had occurred. Furthermore, he saw a case of zoster in each of 35 households in which there were 74 persons who had been in close contact with zoster, and none of whom subsequently developed zoster.

HOPE-SIMPSON (1965) considered that if zoster were caught from a person with chickenpox, then it should be abundant at times when chickenpox was epidemic. On the contrary, he gained the impression from the cases he saw that zoster was less frequent at such times and that perhaps contact with chickenpox conferred some protection against zoster. In addition, over 1,000 persons in household contact with chickenpox in his practice did not develop zoster. Likewise, MILLER and BRUNELL (1970) did not note an increase in the number of their zoster cases corresponding to the seasonal peak of chickenpox. HOPE-SIMPSON (1965) considered that if direct transmission were to occur from zoster patient to zoster patient, persons in the household of zoster patients would be particularly at risk. However, among 318 domiciliary contacts, he noted that no case of zoster was reported.

In view of such evidence it seems that the occurrence of zoster in most instances is not due to the transmission of varicella virus from chickenpox cases or other cases of zoster. It must not be forgotten that if zoster occurs sporadically with no seasonal incidence it is inevitable that sometimes a case of zoster will occur in a contact of chickenpox or zoster by chance but not be causally related to such contact.

E. Special Epidemiological Situations

In most communities both chickenpox and zoster are seen to occur. Zoster has occasionally occurred, however, in isolated communities where chickenpox has never been recorded.

1. Christmas Island

CANTOR (1921) observed that on this island where there was a mixed population fluctuating between 500 and 1,500, zoster was comparatively common, yet chickenpox had been unknown over a period of 20 years. However, the main portion of the population was a "shifting" one, cases of zoster occurring in "casual labourers" from the mainland, and there is no information about the proportion of children in the population susceptible to varicella virus or to what extent they came into contact with the zoster cases.

BRUUSGAARD (1932) in alluding to Cantor's paper, also mentions the Norwegian physician STØREN who in the course of 5 years' practice, in a somewhat isolated district, never saw chickenpox though zoster was by no means infrequent. Of course, an explanation for this could be that chickenpox had occurred many years earlier before STØREN began his observations.

2. Tristan da Cunha

In 1943 the medical officer of this isolated island diagnosed zoster in 3 elderly inhabitants in the population of 220 (WOOLLEY, 1946). Chickenpox had never been known on the island and yet an epidemic of chickenpox did not occur, possibly because zoster cases are not very infectious. Certainly the majority of the population were susceptible, not having experienced chickenpox, because there was an epidemic in 1950. Not all the population developed chickenpox, however, and the apparent partial immunity might be accounted for by a previous epidemic, as postulated by TAYLOR-ROBINSON and TYRRELL (1963), and this in turn could account for the later development of zoster.

X. Pathogenesis

A. Chickenpox

Information on the mode of spread of varicella virus and the development of chickenpox is scanty. THOMSON (1916) exposed susceptible children to patients with typical chickenpox in an open ward without there being direct or intermediate contact. He concluded that the secondary cases of chickenpox which developed did so because of airborne spread of virus. The major source of virus for airborne transmission has not been established. Doubtless transmission can occur from skin lesions, at least while they are in the vesicular stage, since cell-free virus is known to be present (TAYLOR- ROBINSON, 1959). Varicella virus has been isolated from the throat of a single person only on one occasion (GOLD, 1966), there having been other unsuccessful attempts (NELSON and GEME, 1966; CAUNT and SHAW, unpublished). Nevertheless, spread of the virus from the respiratory tract seems indisputable. It was deduced by GORDON and MEADER (1929) who demonstrated the communicability of chickenpox during the 24-hour period preceding the onset of the rash. Similarly, EVANS (1940) observed successful transmission of virus after a single exposure to a case of chickenpox 4 days before the rash occurred. Typical lesions occur in the mucosa of the mouth and pharynx at about the same time as the skin rash appears, but no such oropharyngeal lesions are apparent before this time when the patient is already infectious.

Airborne transmission of varicella virus must result in its inhalation and probable lodgement in the nasopharynx. As HOPE-SIMPSON (1965) postulates, it seems reasonable to suppose that the virus multiplies in the nasopharynx and then produces a primary viraemia. Virus is perhaps removed by the cells of the reticuloendothelial system, within which the virus again multiplies to produce a second much larger viraemia and the scattering of virus to all parts of the body with multiplication especially in the skin and mucous membranes. However, the occurrence of both a primary and a secondary viraemia is speculation. The only evidence for virus being blood-borne comes from the study of necropsy material (CHEATHAM et al., 1956) or of patients who subsequently died (GOLD, 1966).

B. Zoster

DOWNIE (1959) in discussing zoster stated that much concerning its pathogenesis remained unknown. The same statement is true over a decade later although new ideas on the subject have been put forward (HOPE-SIMPSON, 1965).

1. Identity of the Viruses

In considering the pathogenesis of zoster it is necessary to look at the question of whether the virus isolated is the same as that isolated from chickenpox. Clearly the occurrence of zoster after a prior attack of chickenpox could be due to infection with a virus antigenically unlike varicella virus. This, in fact, was a point made many years ago by the proponents of the "dualist" theory (COMBY, 1932); namely that chickenpox and zoster were caused by different agents. However, epidemiological observations, principally that chickenpox occurs in contacts of zoster (p. 55) and the experimental infections previously noted (p. 46), lead one to suppose that the viruses causing the two clinical conditions are the same. This view is strongly supported by various laboratory investigations (p. 13) the results of which show unequivocally that the viruses isolated from chickenpox and zoster patients are antigenically indistinguishable, at least by the techniques that have been used so far. The latter reservation is put forward because quantitative neutralization techniques that are now available have not been used to study this problem, although from the neutralization tests that have been done there is no indication that differences might be revealed.

2. Secondary Antibody Response

The antibody response in zoster (p. 48) is indicative of a secondary response to stimulation by varicella virus in a person who has previously had experience of it. Thus, the antibody titres are greater after zoster than after chickenpox, the response is more rapid than in chickenpox and the class of antibody produced is suggestive of a secondary response (LEONARD et al., 1970). GOLD and GODEK (1965) were not impressed by the more rapid antibody response in zoster. They suggested that an acute-phase serum in zoster is not the same as in chickenpox since the onset of the rash in zoster is not the onset of the disease; the occurrence of pain is indicative of virus activity before this. It seems to us, however, that the same argument might be used in the case of chickenpox. Here virus infection has occurred for at least 10 days before the rash appears and since the spread is haematogenous, antibody-forming cells might have a greater chance of being exposed to the virus in chickenpox than in zoster where the virus is probably often confined to the sensory ganglia and nerves until it reaches the skin.

3. Reinfection or Reactivation of Latent Virus

The argument so far presented is that zoster is due to the growth of varicella virus in a person who has previously been infected with the virus during an attack of chickenpox. Zoster might then occur as a result of reinfection or of reactivation of latent varicella virus, and these possibilities are now considered. There is ample evidence against reinfection by varicella virus as a cause of zoster. The possibility of chickenpox transmitting zoster, or zoster transmitting zoster directly has been discussed (p. 56); it was concluded that if either of these events occurred then they were indeed rare. HOPE-SIMPSON (1965) pointed out that it was necessary to exercise caution before dismissing out of hand the possibility of this sort of transmission because the occasional occurrence of zoster in a contact of zoster was sometimes difficult to refute. However, he adds that it is not possible to found a general hypothesis for the causation of zoster upon a rare event, namely reinfection. This means, therefore, that attention has to be focused on the alternative explanation of reactivation of latent varicella virus. This is an explanation that is probably widely accepted at present.

4. Virus Latency

As pointed out previously (p. 57), it may be difficult to obtain a history of previous chickenpox infection in those who develop zoster, although in the case of zoster occurring in children this may often be obtained. The observations of CANTOR (1921) and WOOLLEY (1946) (p. 58) that in isolated communities zoster occurred but chickenpox was unknown, seem to be the strongest evidence against the theory of virus latency. However, it is not clear if those who suffered from zoster had been born outside the isolated communities and whether they were known not to have had chickenpox. The appearance of "symptomatic" zoster closely following tuberculosis, tumours and injury of the spine, leukaemia, X-ray and immunosuppressive therapy and administration of arsenic suggests the activation of latent virus. Furthermore, in zoster in the elderly there is occasionally incontravertible evidence for prior isolation of the subject from both chickenpox and zoster and when this is so it seems that the recurrent manifestation of a latent virus is the only explanation for the zoster illness.

The observations and reports of some of the earlier workers indicate that the possibility of virus being present in the body in a latent form before the zoster eruption had not occurred to them. HASLUND (1900) noted that zoster might be ushered in with respiratory symptoms and suggested, therefore, that the virus entered the body through the tonsils. He suggested that thereafter it was carried in the blood stream to one or more spinal ganglia and, in certain cases, to the skin also, thus explaining the production of "aberrant" vesicles. Low (1919) suggested that the virus spread from the nose by the olefactory perineural lymphatics to the meninges and cerebrospinal fluid and thence to the spinal ganglia. CHEATHAM (1953) carried out an extensive histological examination of a fatal case of zoster. On the basis of the inclusion bodies observed he proposed that in this case virus had entered the oesophagus, had been transported to the sympathetic ganglion by visceral nerves and had entered the dorsal root ganglion by the white ramus. He considered that the respiratory and gastro-intestinal tracts probably served as portals of virus entry in most cases of zoster. MONTGOMERY (1921) did not appreciate the virus nature of the condition but he was the first to consider nerve transmission, his idea being movement of an agent from and not to the skin. If the agent diffused haematogenously he thought that it would be strange for it to hit one ganglion, or at most two, and if it affected two, that these should be close together on one side of the body. He considered that this might happen in an occasional instance, but not practically every time. He thought it more reasonable to suppose that perhaps due to minor injury the agent entered the nerve terminals in the skin just before the clinical attack of zoster, and ascended to the ganglion of that nerve to cause acute inflammation which in turn caused the skin eruption. VAN ROOYEN and RHODES (1948) and MASSARELLI (1968) considered this theory the most tenable. STERN (1937) reviewed the ideas put forward up to that time and suggested that virus descended in the nerve because in early cases of zoster he found that the skin lesions spread distally along the course of the sensory nerve distribution. This is supported by an observation of LORANT (1968) that prior division of the thoracic sensory nerves appeared to block the spread of a zoster eruption in an area distal to the surgical scar. There seems no doubt, therefore, that varicella virus descends the sensory nerve to the skin, probably from the posterior-root ganglion. The question of how it gets to the ganglion in the first instance is more puzzling. TEAGUE and GOODPASTURE (1923) studied herpes simplex virus in the rabbit. They thought that the virus multiplied in the skin, ascended the spinal nerve to the ganglion and then spread centrifugally back along the nerve and its branches to the skin; they termed their system "experimental herpes zoster". This, of course, followed shortly after MONTGOMERY (1921) had put forward the idea that the agent of zoster spread in the nerves from the skin. The herpes simplex analogy was taken up again by GARLAND (1943) who suggested that, like recurrent herpes simplex infections in man, clinical zoster reflected an activation of a latent varicella virus. These various ideas are brought together by HOPE-SIMPSON (1964, 1965) who provides compelling evidence for varicella virus becoming latent after chickenpox, an aspect not considered by MONTGOMERY (1921). He goes on to point out that the virus has the opportunity to establish itself by the circulatory route in the ganglia during the chickenpox viraemia, a theory now widely held (JOHNSON and MIMS, 1968; JOHNSON, 1968). HOPE-SIMPSON argues, however, that if the haematogenous route is postulated it would be necessary to explain how, out of all the situations in the body, the ganglia only seem to be affected by zoster, and out of all the ganglionic masses in the body the sensory ganglia, almost alone, are affected. This could be most easily explained by passage of virus from the skin and mucosal surfaces during chickenpox to the ganglia via the sensory nerve fibres. It is the sensory ganglia which offer the first opportunity for nuclear lodgement. When, as sometimes occurs, a mixed ganglion is affected by zoster, the motor portion is usually spared and the sensory portion involved. In explaining the precision with which the sensory ganglia are selected, the nerve route demands less special pleading than the haematogenous route. Furthermore, HOPE-SIMPSON presents another argument in favour of the neural route. He noted that the pattern of incidence of zoster on the individual sensory ganglia (Fig. 10) was similar to the distribution of the rash in chickenpox, and may bear a direct relationship to it. An area with dense chickenpox rash may establish more latent virus in the related ganglia, and in return bear more attacks of zoster in later life.

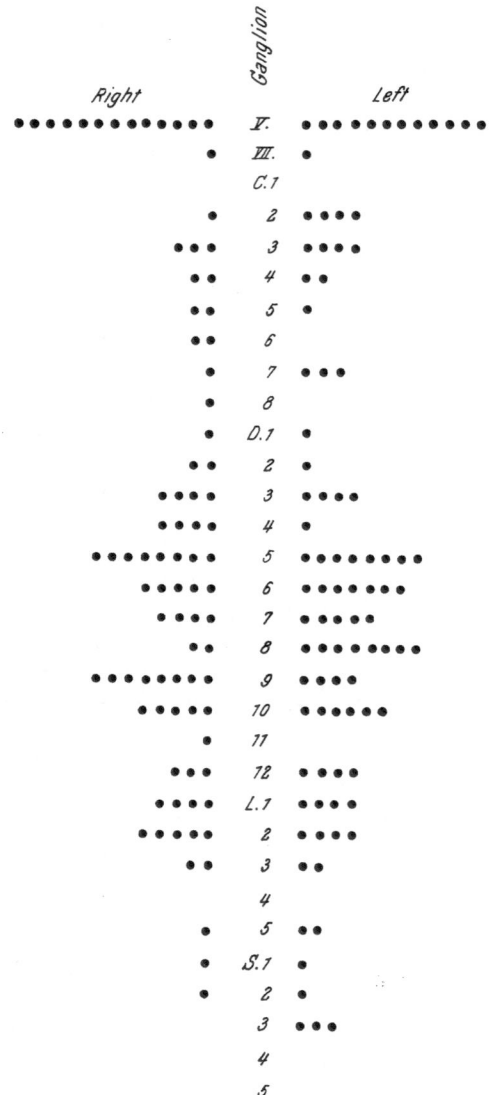

Fig. 10. Distribution of attacks of zoster on individual sensory ganglia. From R. E. Hope-Simpson, Proc. roy. Soc. Med., **58**, 9—20 (1965)

The exact site of latent varicella virus is unknown. If it should be in the posterior root ganglia the only unequivocal evidence regarding its presence there and, in fact, its state of latency would be the isolation of virus in tissue culture from root ganglia, not only in those who have had zoster but more especially in those who have had chickenpox only. However, it may be that virus in a latent form ("provirus" as HOPE-SIMPSON refers to it) would be different from infectious virus and the demonstration of its presence in tissue culture might be more difficult. Certainly, attempts to detect it have not been successful; MEURISSE (1969) failed to isolate varicella virus from the ganglia of the fifth cranial nerves of 66 elderly patients who had died from diseases other than chickenpox and zoster. It is interesting to note that JOHNSON (1940) thought that the presence of degenerating cells adjacent to well preserved ones in a few fragments of dorsal root ganglia, from a patient dying on the third day of a chickenpox eruption, might indicate localization of virus. The search for inclusions in the posterior root ganglia of fatal chickenpox cases has been fruitless or neglected. It may be noted, however, that CHEATHAM et al. (1956) in their case of chickenpox with a zosteriform eruption found inclusion bodies in ganglia other than the one thought to be directly associated with the zosteriform eruption.

The causes of reactivation are a matter for speculation. JUEL-JENSEN (1970) suggests that trauma may be often an exciting cause but the frequency of minor injuries makes it difficult to assess their significance. When zoster follows closely on injury or X-ray to the spine, etc. (p. 60) it seems that these may have been the initial precipitating factors. In many cases of zoster, however, there is no obvious exciting cause. HOPE-SIMPSON (1965) postulates that a decline in antibody titre with advancing age is an important factor. He considers that occasionally non-infectious latent virus reverts to infectious virus. Most often nothing perceptible happens because the virus is neutralized by circulating antibody before it can multiply sufficiently to cause damage. With passage of time antibody declines below a level necessary to inhibit multiplication so that this occurs. Infectious virus then travels down the sensory nerve, causing neuritis and neuralgia, and is released around the sensory nerve endings into the skin to produce the characteristic clusters of zoster vesicles.

If this hypothesis is to be accepted several difficulties require explanation. Firstly, if varicella virus is latent within nerve ganglia how can its reactivation and subsequent spread be influenced by circulating antibody? Perhaps cell-mediated immunity is an important factor and certainly one that requires investigation. Secondly, GIBBS et al. (1970) cite the case of a mother who developed zoster one month after giving birth to twins. The latter did not develop chickenpox following contact with the mother but a 4 year-old sibling did. The authors deduce that the twins received sufficient maternal antibody to protect them but that this antibody did not prevent zoster. It is fair to point out, however, that antibody was not measured and that the twins were given immune serum globulin as a prophylactic measure so that the observation is somewhat difficult to interpret. Thirdly, multiple attacks of zoster occur. Indeed, an attack of zoster does not confer immunity, the likelihood of having a second attack being about as great as having the first (p. 47). If it is postulated that antibody plays an essential part in preventing zoster and that the antibody response after zoster is greater, more persistent and of a different immunoglobulin class than after chickenpox, it would seem that a second attack of zoster would be less likely to occur than a first. Fourthly, if reactivation occurs, why does it lead to zoster and not to chickenpox?

It can only be presumed that the speed of the antibody response, more rapid in zoster than in chickenpox (p. 48), is such as to prevent the widespread haemato-genous distribution of the varicella virus and to keep it localized. It seems, however, that if the antibody response is less rapid or an amount of virus is produced which cannot be completely neutralized, then it "escapes" from the local area of the zoster rash to produce a generalized eruption (p. 41). Indeed, a few scattered vesicles are not infrequently seen in zoster cases. This generalization is likely to be particularly severe where there is underlying malignant disease (p. 41). It seems likely that in such instances the production of circulating varicella virus neutrali-zing antibody is particularly depressed although this has not been proved. Despite such problems, to have a working hypothesis as proposed by HOPE-SIMPSON is valuable since it provides a background against which logical experiments can be done to confirm or refute it.

XI. Prophylaxis

A. Chickenpox

1. Non-Specific Measures

The epidemiological nature of chickenpox is such that there are few practical measures that can be taken for its control. GORDON (1962) points out that indi-vidual notification of cases is not useful and that notification of an unusual case of epidemic occurrence, lest it be due to smallpox, would seem to serve all practical needs. Isolation of patients does little to limit the number of cases because trans-mission of infection is so frequent before the rash is apparent. Further, restriction of susceptible persons exposed to chickenpox, for a period equal to the longest incubation period of 21 days, is outmoded. However, there is a clear case for isolating persons with severe blood dyscrasias or those on immunosuppressive drugs. Attempts to prevent spread of infection by the use of ultraviolet irradiation (McKHANN et al., 1938; GREENE et al., 1941; WELLS et al., 1942; McMATH and HUSSAIN, 1960) and triethylene glycol vapour (BAHLKE et al., 1949) are of no practical value.

2. Immunization

a) Active Immunization

Chickenpox is generally a mild disease. It is, therefore, debatable whether an effort to protect individual persons is worthwhile. It would seem to be so for certain poor-risk patients but in such cases prevention is best achieved by passive immunization (see p. 65). Prevention of chickenpox on a widespread scale is another consideration. The need for a vaccine has been discussed by WELLER (1967). If zoster is a long term sequel of chickenpox then effective vaccination against the latter would also eliminate zoster. Since about half of those who reach the age of 85 years have suffered zoster (HOPE-SIMPSON, 1965), chickenpox prophylaxis is probably worthy of consideration for this reason alone.

Mention has already been made (p. 46) of the vaccination of children with vesicle fluid from chickenpox and zoster patients and their purported subsequent immunity. GREENTHAL (1926) used the procedure on 36 persons, of whom 19 had a local reaction. These vaccinated persons did not develop chickenpox after exposure to the disease, while some of the unvaccinated population did, which suggests that protection had been achieved. It is difficult to assess whether this was really so, however, because chickenpox did not develop in those who were unsuccessfully vaccinated. GULÁCSY (1933) considered that immunization was successful even though a local skin reaction did not occur; this seems doubtful. WESSELHOEFT (1944) has given an account of such inoculation procedures which would seem to be of very limited practical value and have not been used for more than a quarter of a century.

Alternatively, virus produced in tissue culture in the laboratory might be used as a vaccine. There is no indication that varicella virus comprises more than a single immunological type and, therefore, a vaccine prepared from virus isolated from any case of disease, whether it be chickenpox or zoster, should be effective. It is conceivable that the use of a live, attenuated virus vaccine would prevent clinical chickenpox but might result in virus becoming latent and being manifest as zoster in later life. This problem could be avoided by using a vaccine which contained killed viral material. A major difficulty seems to be the present inability to obtain virus in sufficient quantity free from cells. On the other hand, it may be unnecessary to make efforts to produce infectious virus in tissue culture. It is known (p. 26) that although fluids from varicella virus-infected cultures rarely contain infectious virus particles they do contain many non-infectious particles. Perhaps these are capable of stimulating neutralizing antibody. In this respect, the brief report by IOULEV et al. (1969) is interesting. It seems that they used fluids from the thirty-fifth tissue-culture passage of varicella virus to inoculate children, some of whom developed a rise in complement-fixing antibody.

b) Passive Immunization

WEECH (1924), GORDON and MEADER (1929), GUNN (1932) and LEWIS et al. (1937) used early convalescent-phase sera in attempts to prevent chickenpox in contacts but the method was never sufficiently dependable to be of use in epidemic control. Subsequently, γ-globulin has been used by a number of workers but in some instances the observations are difficult to interpret because the studies were uncontrolled (GREENBERG, 1947; FUNKHOUSER, 1948). SCHAEFFER and TOOMEY (1948) in a study of chickenpox contacts, some of whom were given γ-globulin, did not find that this prevented or ameliorated the disease. TRIMBLE (1957), however, considered that there probably was attenuation of disease but the number of patients he studied was too small to draw definite conclusions. ROSS (1962) was the first to report a large controlled study of the effect of γ-globulin in contacts. He did not note any preventive effect but did conclude that chickenpox could be modified with relatively large doses; children treated in this way had fewer skin vesicles and lower temperatures. BODEY et al. (1964) gave 6 of 12 leukaemic patients γ-globulin shortly after exposure to chickenpox; compared to the untreated patients, the course of the disease in those treated was milder with fewer vesicles. On the other hand, ARNOULT and RENDTORFF (1962), SCHAFFER (1965) and SHAW and GROSSMAN (1966) found γ-globulin unreliable in protecting susceptible contacts. It seems likely that the conflicting results are a reflection of the amount of antibody in the various preparations used. It is clear from previous work (p. 48) that antibody of the greatest titre and, indeed, antibody of a different class (LEONARD *et al.*, 1970) is to be found in zoster convalescent-phase sera rather than in chickenpox sera. ABRAMSON (1944), unaware of this fact, administered zoster convalescent-phase serum to chickenpox contacts in an attempt to demonstrate a relationship between the two clinical conditions. He observed chickenpox in 4 of 6 untreated children but in only 1 of 8 treated children. A further, and even more convincing demonstration of chickenpox prophylaxis has been reported by BRUNELL *et al.* (1969) who used γ-globulin prepared from donors who were recovering from zoster. In this double-blind study, the administration of a 2 ml dose of zoster immune globulin to susceptible children within 72 hours of their exposure to chickenpox prevented the disease, whereas it occurred in 6 siblings likewise exposed who received normal human serum γ-globulin. All the reports mentioned are concerned with intramuscular inoculations. However, RUSTI (1957) considered that chickenpox convalescent-phase serum put on the eyes of children protected them against chickenpox. There are no other reports to confirm this assertion.

Indications for prophylactic therapy are perhaps beyond the scope of this review. However, it would seem reasonable to use γ-globulin, prepared from sera of those recovering from zoster, particularly in persons receiving immunosuppressive therapy and in those with blood dyscrasias, who have been exposed to chickenpox. IRIARTE *et al.* (1965) have administered γ-globulin to such patients with malignant disease but it is not possible to assess the value of the therapy they used since the study was uncontrolled. McDONAGH (1966) points out that the serious chickenpox illness which may occur in adults is not an indication for the routine use of γ-globulin in contacts but perhaps only in poor-risk patients.

3. Antiviral Drugs

RAPP (1964) treated human embryo lung cells with N-methyl-isatin-thiosemi-carbazone (Marboran) at a concentration of 1 μg/ml (about 5 μM) and then infected them with varicella virus. He concluded that this drug did not affect plaque formation by the virus although this might have been due to the fact that free infectious virus was not liberated from these cells. CAUNT (1967) used human thyroid tissue cultures from which some virus can be released. She found that Marboran treatment (20 μM) suppressed the amount of virus that could be freed from the cells and that the degree of suppression was related to the concentration used. However, from a practical point of view it does not seem that the drug is valuable. In a small prophylactic clinical trial of Marboran, REED *et al.* (1966), using a regimen that had been employed successfully in smallpox (BAUER, 1965), did not observe a difference in the number of clinical cases or in the severity of illness between the treated and control groups.

BRUCE (1966) gave N', N'-anhydrobis (β-hydroxyethyl) biguanide hydrochloride (abitylguanide; ABOB; Virugon) to family contacts of chickenpox cases but failed to show that it protected them.

B. Zoster

Because of its sporadic, non-epidemic nature the prevention of zoster is difficult. However, it might be possible to boost the titre of neutralizing antibody in adults by using a varicella virus vaccine. A controlled vaccine trial in an adult population would be worthwhile since it might provide a means of prevention and at the same time help to confirm or refute the idea that zoster is due to a waning level of varicella virus neutralizing antibody. It is conceivable that a varicella virus vaccine might be used more profitably in this way than in attempts to eliminate chickenpox from the younger generation.

XII. Treatment

A. Chickenpox

It is not within the scope of this review to consider the supportive therapy that is given to patients suffering from severe attacks of chickenpox. However, some of the other measures that have been used are worth mentioning. It would seem logical to use γ-globulin, preferably zoster immune globulin, in patients with severe chickenpox particularly where this complicates an underlying disease such as leukaemia. The severity of the chickenpox might be due to a prolonged viraemia which could be diminished by γ-globulin treatment. In this respect, LOEBL and TAYLOR (1966) thought that γ-globulin from convalescent chickenpox patients was helpful in the treatment of a severe case of chickenpox.

CURWEN et al. (1963) in a controlled trial attempted to determine the therapeutic value of the antiviral compound abitylguanide. They found that the duration of fever was shorter in the treated patients than in those in the control group but that the difference was of borderline significance only; they were not able to assess accurately whether the rash was modified by the drug. MENUT et al. (1964) considered that the compound was of no value. It is not possible to assess whether 5-iodo-2'-deoxyuridine was beneficial in the case of corneal chickenpox in which it was used (CAIRNS, 1964). KIBRICK and KATZ (1970) used 0.5 per cent IUDR ointment to treat 4 patients with early varicella infections. The ointment was ineffective in modifying the eruptions. However, the concentration of IUDR was less than that used by JUEL-JENSEN (1970) for the treatment of zoster and also the substance was not incorporated in dimethyl sulphoxide (p. 68). It is of interest that chickenpox has been recorded in leukaemic patients under treatment with cytosine arabinoside (SELIGMAN and ROSNER, 1970). The doses used, however, were probably insufficient to have had an anti-viral effect.

B. Zoster

Protamide, a proteolytic enzyme from pig stomach, has frequently been used in the treatment of zoster, but BOUNDY and BAMFORD (1968) in a controlled trial convincingly demonstrated its uselessness. Equally without benefit is the use of X-ray therapy (RHYS-LEWIS, 1965). Steroids have been administered over a short period (PESTEL, 1961; ELLIOTT, 1964; HOPE-SIMPSON, 1967) and EAGLSTEIN et al. (1970) demonstrated in a double-blind trial that steroid therapy did not affect the rate of skin healing but it did shorten the post-herpetic neuralgia particularly in those less than 60 years old. The use of broad-spectrum antibiotics has been thought by some to be of value in relieving pain and in rapidly healing the lesions (BINDER and STUBBS, 1949; MARAN et al., 1967). However, these were impressions gained in treating a few patients and have not been borne out in more thorough controlled trials (CARTER, 1951; KASS et al., 1952).

Several other approaches to the treatment of zoster are now considered. The relief of pain and the modification and lack of progression of skin lesions in zoster patients treated with γ-globulin has been reported by GROS (1952), WEINTRAUB (1955), RODARTE and WILLIAMS (1956), LEA and TAYLOR (1958) and BREFFEILH (1961). On the other hand, EPSTEIN and ALLINGTON (1957) considered that such treatment was valueless. Unfortunately, all these reports are based on observations made on treated patients only and, therefore, the possible beneficial effects of γ-globulin cannot be assessed, particularly since the γ-globulin preparations used were of unknown potency.

SCHERSTEN (1959), WILKINSON (1962) and DUPERRAT (1963) treated zoster patients with the antiviral compound abitylguanide and suggested that the lesions healed and the pain disappeared more rapidly than was usual. However, the opposite impression was gained in another study (G. P. Clinical Trials, 1965). There certainly seems no point in considering this drug further.

RAWLS et al. (1964) found that IUDR in concentrations of 5 μg/ml greatly diminished the cytopathic effect of varicella virus in human diploid fibroblasts, being effective when the cultures were treated even as long as 3 days after challenge with the virus. They suggested that the compound might find some use in cases of serious disease. CALABRESI (1965) attempted to assess the value of systemic IUDR therapy in patients with neoplastic disorders complicated by zoster, but was unable to come to a definite conclusion principally because of the severity of the underlying disease. WALTUCH and SACKS (1968) treated a single case of Hodgkin's disease in which zoster had developed and was complicated by a generalized rash. They gave IUDR systematically, but on the basis of a single case it is not possible to interpret the apparent excellent response as being due to the antimetabolite. McCALLUM (1963) treated six patients suffering from trigeminal zoster with a topical application of 0.1 per cent IUDR solution. While he thought that the response was encouraging, he was clearly not able to come to a definite conclusion and so he and his colleagues (McCALLUM et al., 1964) organized a double-blind trial to determine whether topical application of 0.1 per cent IUDR was effective. The severity and duration of pain and the duration of the eruption was not reduced in the treated zoster patients. On the other hand, JUEN-JENSEN (1970) also carried out a double-blind trial and reported that the topical application of 5 per cent IUDR incorporated in dimethyl sulphoxide resulted in more rapid healing of zoster lesions, and a shortening of the duration of pain. Continuous application of a 40 per cent solution of IUDR in dimethyl sulphoxide gave even better results; the duration of pain was reduced from more than a month to less than 3 days. The results were particularly striking in those persons aged 60 years or more. Perhaps these results are due to the greater concentration of IUDR used and a greater penetration of the antimetabolite when it is mixed with dimethyl sulphoxide.

XIII. Laboratory Diagnosis

Laboratory help is not required for the diagnosis of typical clinical cases of chickenpox or zoster. Various laboratory procedures are available, however, for assessing atypical cases, or in the differential diagnosis of smallpox which may on occasion prove difficult (THOMPSON, 1967). The earlier use of rabbits (SALMON, 1905) and monkeys (PARK, 1902) which responded to inoculation of smallpox material but not of chickenpox, has been superseded by other methods.

A. Electron Microscopy

In the differential diagnosis between chickenpox and smallpox the morphology of the virus particles negatively stained with phosphotungstic acid and viewed in the electron microscope will distinguish herpesvirus particles from those of the poxvirus group (CRUICKSHANK et al., 1966; p. 8). Vesicle fluid is the best source of virus but pustule fluid or crusts may be used. The result of such an examination can be available in about 30 minutes and this is the quickest way of excluding smallpox but does not distinguish between the herpesviruses. ESIRI and TOMLINSON (1971) make the point that electron microscopy is probably more useful than virus culture for examining post-mortem tissue since varicella virus is particularly labile.

B. Histopathology

Multinucleate giant epithelial cells and intranuclear inclusions may be seen in a Giemsa-stained smear of a scraping from the base of an early vesicle (p. 38). These findings are characteristic of the changes produced by the herpesviruses (BLANK et al., 1951) and help when the diagnosis of smallpox has to be considered. The same changes may be observed also in skin biopsy material, and similar changes have been described in smears of oral mucosa (COOKE, 1960; 1963). Examination of the sputum may be worthwhile in those patients who develop pneumonia apparently as a complication of chickenpox; WILLIAMS and CAPERS (1959) considered that the occurrence of intranuclear inclusions in cells in the sputum of a patient with chickenpox pneumonia confirmed the diagnosis.

C. Gel Diffusion

Vesicle fluid may be used in gel-diffusion tests (pp. 15, 48) (TAYLOR-ROBINSON and RONDLE, 1959) in the same way as described by DUMBELL and NIZAMUDDIN (1959) for the rapid diagnosis of smallpox. The time required for such tests may be reduced from 2—3 hours to 30 minutes by subjecting the immunodiffusion slides to electrophoresis (NETTER and SIBILAT, 1968). MACRAE et al. (1969) reported that moist tops of lesions, crusts or scabs were also suitable as antigen, but not dried smears of vesicle fluid. DAYAN et al. (1964) successfully used an extract of skin removed at autopsy. A human convalescent zoster serum known to give rapid and easily visible precipitation with chickenpox or zoster vesicle fluids but not with vesicle fluid from herpes simplex virus cases should be used.

D. Detection of Virus

Virus may be isolated in tissue culture from vesicle fluid provided that this is taken early in the course of the disease. Isolation of virus is most certain within 72 hours of onset of the rash but occasionally may be accomplished as late as 6 days (TAYLOR-ROBINSON, 1959; GÉDER et al., 1963; MACRAE et al., 1969) or even later in the case of patients with underlying neoplastic diseases. Vesicle fluid should be inoculated into primary monolayer cultures of human embryo fibroblasts, human thyroid cells or into cultures of semi-continuous strains of human diploid fibroblasts, such as WI 38 cells (p. 21). Other cells may be used but these will generally not be as sensitive as those listed for the isolation of the virus. Cytopathic changes will not usually be visible before 48 hours and in some cases may not appear until 7 to 9 days after inoculation; or they may even require subculture of cells to fresh monolayers before they are obvious (HERRMANN, 1967). The cytopathic change usually remains in focal areas and extends only slowly. This serves to distinguish it from the change produced by herpes simplex virus which rapidly (24 to 48 hours) involves the whole tissue-culture monolayer. To exclude herpes simplex virus infection it is also wise to inoculate the chorio-allantoic membranes of 10 to 12 day-old fertile eggs, which are insensitive to varicella virus (p. 34). A more positive identification of the isolate may be made by a neutralization test using either acute and convalescent-phase sera from a case of chickenpox or zoster, or specific antisera produced in laboratory animals, such as the rabbit antiserum described by MARTOS et al. (1970). Alternatively, the direct or indirect immunofluorescence technique may be used with acute and convalescent-phase sera from a case of zoster (WELLER and COONS, 1964) or hyperimmune sera made in monkeys (SCHMIDT et al., 1965 b) or rabbits (KISSLING et al., 1968).

DAYAN et al. (1964) used an indirect immunofluorescence method to detect virus in sections of lung removed at autopsy; they observed bright fluorescence of intranuclear inclusion bodies. ESIRI and TOMLINSON (1972) used immunofluorescence to detect viral antigen in post-mortem nerve tissue; they considered the direct technique was best because it gave less non-specific staining.

E. Serology

When vesicle fluid is not available or isolation of the virus fails serological tests on the patient's serum may be of help.

Complement-fixation tests (pp. 14, 48) may be performed using antigens prepared in tissue culture (SCHMIDT et al., 1964; BRUNELL and CASEY, 1964; CAUNT and TAYLOR-ROBINSON, 1964). Antibody is detectable 5 to 7 days after the onset of the rash in chickenpox but in zoster it is often detectable on the 1st or 2nd day of the illness. In both diseases it reaches its maximum 2 to 3 weeks after the onset and then declines slowly over a period of 6 months to 2 years. The presence of such complement-fixing antibodies indicates, therefore, recent experience of varicella virus, although it should be noted that a rise in the titre of antibody to varicella virus may occur also in the course of primary herpes simplex virus infections (p. 17) (KAPSENBERG, 1964; SVEDMYR, 1965; SCHMIDT et al., 1969).

Neutralization tests (pp. 16, 48) may be done as described by SCHMIDT *et al.* (1969) or by CAUNT and SHAW (1969) with cell-free virus prepared in primary cultures of human thyroid cells (CAUNT and TAYLOR-ROBINSON, 1964) or in cultures of human diploid fibroblasts (BRUNELL, 1967 b). Neutralizing antibody titres probably reach their maximum at about the same time as those of complement-fixing antibodies, but neutralizing antibodies persist much longer and, therefore, their presence has not the same diagnostic significance as the presence of complement-fixing antibodies in indicating recent infection.

In summary, the procedure used for diagnosis will obviously depend to some extent upon the facilities of the laboratory and any of the techniques described may be used. However, of the diagnostic methods discussed, MACRAE *et al.* (1969) found that electron microscopy was the most efficient. Herpesvirus particles were found in 31 of 32 instances where varicella virus infection was suspected. In the one failure, a gel-diffusion test and culture of virus were successful. However, each of these methods alone was less successful since a definite line of precipitation occurred in only 10 of 30 tests and typical cytopathic effects were observed in only 11 of 16 virus isolation attempts. Where electron microscopy facilities are not available or this technique fails, the next most rapid diagnostic procedure, providing an answer in a few hours, is a gel-diffusion test although clearly this may be unsuccessful. An attempt to culture the virus by inoculation of tissue cultures is worthwhile only if vesicle fluid is available and it may be a few days before cytopathic effects are visible. As a further alternative, providing a less rapid diagnosis, the patient's sera may be examined in a complement-fixation test for a four-fold or greater rise in the titre of antibody to varicella virus.

Acknowledgment

We wish to thank Dr. Janet S. F. Niven of the National Institute for Medical Research, London, for her help in the interpretation of the cytopathic effects of varicella virus *in vitro*, and Mr. M. R. Young, also of the National Institute for Medical Research, who carried out the short wave ultraviolet light absorption microscopy. We thank Mrs. J. D. Almeida for the electron micrograph, the National Foundation and the International Medical Congress, Ltd., New York for permission to use Figs. 8 and 9, and Dr. R. E. Hope-Simpson for Fig. 10. Finally, we thank Professor A. W. Downie and Dr. D. A. J. Tyrrell for their constructive criticism of the manuscript, and Mrs. E. Sparrow and Mrs. P. Moody for typing it.

References

ABRAMSON, A. W.: Varicella and herpes zoster: an experiment. Brit. med. J. **1**, 812—813 (1944).

ACHONG, B. G., and E. V. MEURISSE: Observations on the fine structure and replication of varicella virus in cultivated human amnion cells. J. gen. Virol. **3**, 305—308 (1968).

ADKISSON, M. A.: Herpes zoster in a newborn premature infant. J. Pediat. **66**, 956—958 (1965).

AITKEN, R. S., and R. T. BRAIN: Facial palsy and infection with zoster virus. Lancet **1**, 19—22 (1933).

ALLEN, F. M. B.: Varicella and herpes zoster in the same patient. Brit. med. J. **2**, 115 (1944).

ALMEIDA, J. D., A. F. HOWATSON, and M. G. WILLIAMS: Morphology of varicella (chickenpox) virus. Virology 16, 353—355 (1962).

AMIES, C. R.: The elementary bodies of varicella and their agglutination in pure suspension by the serum of chickenpox patients. Lancet 1, 1015—1017 (1933).

AMIES, C. R.: The elementary bodies of zoster and their serological relationship to those of varicella. Brit. J. exp. Path. 15, 314—320 (1934).

ANDREWES, C. H.: Viruses of Vertebrates. London: Bailliere, Tindall and Cox, 1964.

ANDREWES, C. H., and H. G. PEREIRA: Viruses of Vertebrates, 2nd edition. London: Bailliere, Tindall and Cox, 1967.

APPELBAUM, E., S. I. KREPS, and A. SUNSHINE: Herpes zoster encephalitis. Amer. J. Med. 32, 25—31 (1962).

APPELBAUM, E., M. H. RACHELSON, and V. B. DOLGOPOL: Varicella encephalitis. Amer. J. Med. 15, 223—230 (1953).

ARAGÃO, H. DE B.: Estudos sobre Alastrim. Mem. Inst. Osw. Cruz. 3, 309—319 (1911).

ARMSTRONG, J. A., and J. S. F. NIVEN: Histochemical observations on cellular and virus nucleic acids. Nature (Lond.) 180, 1335—1336 (1957).

ARMSTRONG, R. W., M. J. GURWITH, D. WADDELL, and T. C. MERIGAN: Cutaneous interferon production in patients with Hodgkin's disease and other cancers infected with varicella or vaccinia. New Engl. J. Med. 283, 1182—1187 (1970).

ARMSTRONG, R. W., and T. C. MERIGAN: Varicella zoster virus: interferon production and comparative interferon sensitivity in human cell cultures. J. gen. Virol. 12, 53—54 (1971).

ARNOULT, M. B., and R. C. RENDTORFF: Notes on a trial of low doses of gamma-globulin against chickenpox during an outbreak. Memphis med. J. 37, 69—71 (1962).

ARTENSTEIN, M. S., and L. WEINSTEIN: Simultaneous infection with the viruses of chickenpox and measles. J. Pediat. 62, 156—158 (1963).

AULA, P.: Chromosome breaks in leukocytes of chickenpox patients. Preliminary communication. Hereditas 49, 451—453 (1963).

AULA, P.: Chromosomes and viral infections. Lancet 1, 720—721 (1964).

BACON, G. E., W. J. OLIVER, and B. A. SHAPIRO: Factors contributing to severity of herpes zoster in children. J. Pediat. 67, 768—771 (1965).

BÄRENSPRUNG, VON: Pemphigus. Febris vesiculosa et bullosa — Schälblattern. Ann. Charité — Krankenh. Berl. 10, 55—122 (1862).

BAHLKE, A. M., H. F. SILVERMAN, and H. S. INGRAHAM: Effect of ultra-violet irradiation of classrooms on spread of mumps and chickenpox in large rural central schools. Amer. J. publ. Hlth 39, 1321—1330 (1949).

BAMFORD, J. A. C., and C. A. P. BOUNDY: The natural history of herpes zoster (shingles). Med. J. Aust. 1, 524—528 (1968).

BARNETT, C. H.: The relationship between herpes zoster and varicella. Med. Press (Lond.) 223, 126—128 (1950).

BAUER, D. J.: Clinical experience with the antiviral drug Marboran (1-methylisatin 3-thiosemicarbazone). Ann. N. Y. Acad. Sci. 130, 110—117 (1965).

BEALE, A. J., and G. CHRISTOFINIS: Growth of RK 13 cells. Symposium international sur la standardisation des vaccines contre la rougeole et la serologie de la rubéole, Lyon. pp. 103—104 (1964).

BECKER, P., J. L. MELNICK, and H. D. MAYOR: A morphologic comparison between the developmental stages of herpes zoster and human cytomegalovirus. Exp. molec. Path. 4, 11—23 (1965).

BEDSON, S. P., and J. O. W. BLAND: Complement-fixation with filterable viruses and their antisera. Brit. J. exp. Path. 10, 393—404 (1929).

BENYESH-MELNICK, M., H. F. STICH, F. RAPP, and T. C. HSU: Viruses and mammalian chromosomes. III. Effect of herpes zoster virus on human embryonal lung cultures. Proc. Soc. exp. Biol. (N. Y.) 117, 546—549 (1964).

BINDER, M. L., and L. E. STUBBS: Treatment of herpes zoster with aureomycin. J. Amer. med. Ass. 141, 1050—1051 (1949).

BIRKS, D. A.: Herpes zoster ophthalmicus in an 8 year old child. Brit. J. Ophthal. 47, 60—61 (1963).

BLANK, H., C. F. BURGOON, G. D. BALDRIDGE, P. L. MCCARTHY, and F. URBACH: Cytologic smears in diagnosis of herpes simplex, herpes zoster, and varicella. J. Amer. med. Ass. **146**, 1410—1412 (1951).

BLANK, H., L. L. CORIELL, and T. F. M. SCOTT: Human skin grafted on the chorioallantois of the chick embryo for virus cultivation. Proc. Soc. exp. Biol. (N. Y.) **69**, 341—345 (1948).

BLANK, H., and G. RAKE: "Viral and Rickettsial Diseases of the Skin, Eye and Mucous Membranes of Man". 1st Ed. pp. 71—96. Boston: Little, Brown and Co. (1955).

BLATT, M. L., M. ZELDES, and A. F. STEIN: Chickenpox following contact with herpes zoster. Report of two minor epidemics. J. Lab. clin. Med. **25**, 951—955 (1939—1940).

BODEY, G., E. MCKELVEY, and M. KARON: Chickenpox in leukemic patients— factors in prognosis. Pediatrics **34**, 562—564 (1964).

BÓKAY, J. VON: Über den ätiologischen Zusammenhang der Varizellen mit gewissen Fällen von Herpes Zoster. Wien. klin. Wschr. **22**, 1323—1326 (1909).

BÓKAY, J. VON: Über die Identität der Ätiologie der Schafblattern und einzelner Fälle von Herpes zoster. Jb. Kinderheilk. **89**, 380—394 (1919).

BÓKAY, J. VON: Über die Herpes-zoster-Varizellen-Frage. Jb. Kinderheilk. **105**, 8—23 (1924).

BÓKAY, J. VON: Gürtelrose und Windpocken. Jb. Kinderheilk. **119**, 127—160 (1928).

BONAR, B. E., and C. J. PEARSALL: Herpes zoster in the new-born. Amer. J. Dis. Child. **44**, 398—402 (1932).

BOUGHTON, C. R.: Varicella-zoster in Sydney. II. Neurological complications of varicella. Med. J. Aust. **2**, 444—447 (1966 a).

BOUGHTON, C. R.: Varicella-zoster in Sydney. III. Herpes zoster and complications. Med. J. Aust. **2**, 502—504 (1966 b).

BOUNDY, C. A. P., and J. A. C. BAMFORD: Treatment of herpes zoster with "Protamide". Med. J. Aust. **1**, 528—531 (1968).

BRAIN, R. T.: The relationship between the viruses of zoster and varicella as demonstrated by the complement-fixation reaction. Brit. J. exp. Path. **14**, 67—73 (1933).

BRAIN, W. R.: Zoster, varicella and encephalitis. Brit. med. J. **1**, 81—84 (1931).

BREFFEILH, L. A.: The use of gammaglobulin in the treatment of herpes zoster and herpes simplex. J. Louisiana med. Soc. **113**, 502—506 (1961).

BREWER, T. F.: Congenital varicella with primary varicella pneumonia. Calif. Med. **92**, 350—353 (1960).

BRIGHT, R.: Reports of Medical Cases. London; **2**, pt. 1, 383 (1831).

British Medical Journal: Any Questions? Recurrence of herpes zoster. **2**, 39 (1968).

BRODKIN, R. H.: Zoster causing varicella: current dangers of contagion without isolation. Arch. Derm. **88**, 322—324 (1963).

BRODY, I. A., and R. H. WILKINS: Ramsay Hunt syndrome. Arch. Neurol. (Chic.) **18**, 583—589 (1968).

BROSTOFF, J.: Diaphragmatic paralysis after herpes zoster. Brit. med. J., **2**, 1571—1572 (1966).

BROWDER, J., and J. A. DE VEER: Herpes zoster: a surgical procedure for the treatment of postherpetic neuralgia. Ann. Surg. **130**, 622—636 (1949).

BRUCE, R.: Attempted chickenpox prophylaxis with Virugon in contacts. J. Coll. gen. Practit. **11**, 341—343 (1966).

BRUNELL, P. A.: Placental transfer of varicella-zoster antibody. Pediatrics **38**, 1034—1038 (1966).

BRUNELL, P. A.: Varicella-zoster infections in pregnancy. J. Amer. med. Ass. **199**, 315—317 (1967 a).

BRUNELL, P. A.: Separation of infectious varicella-zoster virus from human embryonic lung fibroblasts. Virology **31**, 732—734 (1967 b).

BRUNELL, P. A.: Personal communication (1968).

BRUNELL, P. A., and H. L. CASEY: Crude tissue culture antigen for determination of varicella-zoster complement fixing antibody. Publ. Hlth Rep. (Wash.) **79**, 839—842 (1964).

BRUNELL, P. A., L. H. MILLER, and F. LOVEJOY: Zoster in children. Amer. J. Dis. Child. **115**, 432—437 (1968).

BRUNELL, P. A., A. ROSS, L. H. MILLER, and B. KUO: Prevention of varicella by zoster immune globulin. New Engl. J. Med. **280**, 1191—1194 (1969).

BRUUSGAARD, E.: The mutual relation between zoster and varicella. Brit. J. Derm. Syph. **44**,1—24 (1932).

BUDDINGH, G. J.: Infection of the chorio-allantois of the chick embryo as a diagnostic test for variola. Amer. J. Hyg. **28**, 130—137 (1938).

BULLOWA, J. G. M., and S. M. WISHIK: Complications of varicella. I. Their occurrence among 2,534 patients. Amer. J. Dis. Child. **49**, 923—926 (1935).

BURGOON, C. F. JR., J. S. BURGOON, and G. D. BALDRIDGE: The natural history of herpes zoster. J. Amer. med. Ass. **164**, 265—269 (1957).

BURNET, F. M., and D. LUSH: The propagation of the virus of infectious ectromelia of mice in the developing egg. J. Path. Bact. **43**, 105—120 (1936).

CAIRNS, J. E.: Varicella of the cornea treated with 5-iodo-2'-deoxyuridine. Brit. J. Ophthal. **48**, 288—289 (1964).

CALABRESI, P.: Clinical studies with systemic administration of antimetabolites of pyrimidine nucleosides in viral infections. Ann. N. Y. Acad. Sci. **130**, 192—208 (1965).

CAMPBELL, R. M.: Varicella and herpes zoster, with a report of three illustrated cases. Brit. J. Child. Dis. **38**, 91—98 (1941).

CANTOR, S. J.: Herpes and varicella. Brit. med. J. **2**, 508 (1921).

CARTER, A. B.: Investigation into the effects of aureomycin and chloramphenicol in herpes zoster. Brit. med. J. **1**, 987—991 (1951).

CAUNT, A. E.: Growth of varicella-zoster virus in human thyroid tissue cultures. Lancet **2**, 982—983 (1963).

CAUNT, A. E.: The effect of Marboran on the growth of varicella virus in tissue culture. Fifth International Congress of Chemotherapy, Vienna, 313—317 (1967).

CAUNT, A. E.: The growth of varicella-zoster virus in tissue fragments. Brit. J. exp. Path. **50**, 26—31 (1969).

CAUNT, A. E., C. J. M. RONDLE, and A. W. DOWNIE: The soluble antigens of varicella-zoster virus produced in tissue culture. J. Hyg. (Lond.) **59**, 249—258 (1961).

CAUNT, A. E., and D. G. SHAW: Neutralization tests with varicella-zoster virus. J. Hyg. (Lond.) **67**, 343—352 (1969).

CAUNT, A. E., and D. TAYLOR-ROBINSON: Cell-free varicella-zoster virus in tissue culture. J. Hyg. (Lond.) **62**, 413—424 (1964).

CHARLES, R. H. G.: Post-varicella polyneuritis. Brit. med. J. **1**, 908 (1965).

CHEATHAM, W. J.: The relation of heretofore unreported lesions to pathogenesis of herpes zoster. Amer. J. Path. **29**, 401—411 (1953).

CHEATHAM, W. J., T. H. WELLER, T. F. DOLAN, and J. C. DOWER: Varicella: report of two fatal cases with necropsy, virus isolation and serologic studies. Amer. J. Path. **32**, 1015—1035 (1956).

CHERNIAVSKAIA, R. I., N. I. A. CHINIAKOVA, and R. I. ZAKASHANSKAIA: Varicella meningo-encephalomyelitis with fatal outcome in a 7½-year old child. Vop. Okhrany Materin. Dets. **10**, 85—88 (1965).

CHRISTENSEN, P. E., H. SCHMIDT, H. O. BANG, V. ANDERSEN, B. JORDAL, and O. JENSEN: An epidemic of measles in Southern Greenland, 1951. Acta med. scand. **144**, 430—449 (1953).

CHRISTIE, A. B.: Infectious Diseases; Epidemiology and Clinical Practice. Edinburgh: Livingstone, 1969.

CHUN, T., D. S. ALEXANDER, A. M. BRYANS, and M. D. HAUST: Chromosomal studies in children with mumps, chickenpox, measles and measles vaccination. Canad. med. Ass. J. **94**, 126—129 (1966).

CLAUDY, W. D.: Pneumonia associated with varicella. Review of the literature and report of a fatal case with autopsy. Arch. intern. Med. **80**, 185—192 (1947).

COLE, R., and A. G. KUTTNER: The problem of the etiology of herpes zoster. J. exp. Med. **42**, 799—820 (1925).

COMBY, J.: La varicelle et le zona. J. Méd. Paris 52, 599 (1932).

COOK, M. L., and J. G. STEVENS: Labile coat: reason for noninfectious cell-free varicella-zoster virus in culture. J. Virol. 2, 1458—1464 (1968).

COOK, M. L., and J. G. STEVENS: Replication of varicella-zoster virus in cell culture: an ultrastructural study. J. Ultrastruct. Res. 32, 334—350 (1970).

COOKE, B. E. D.: Epithelial smears in diagnosis of herpes simplex and herpes zoster affecting the oral mucosa. Brit. dent. J. 109, 83—96 (1960).

COOKE, B. E. D.: Exfoliative cytology in evaluating oral lesions. J. dent. Res. (Suppl.) 42, 343—347 (1963).

COORAY, M. P. M.: Ten cases of fatal haemorrhagic chickenpox in Ceylon. J. trop. Med. Hyg. 68, 174—176 (1965).

COUNTER, C. E., and B. J. KORN: Herpes zoster in the newborn associated with congenital blindness. Arch. Pediat. 67, 397—399 (1950).

COWDRY, E. V.: The problem of intranuclear inclusions in virus diseases. Arch. Path. 18, 527—542 (1934).

COWIE, J. M.: Herpes zoster and varicella (Letter to Editor). Brit. med. J. 1, 642 (1925).

CRANDELL, R. A.: The herpes virus group. Amer. J. vet. Res. 28, 577—582 (1967).

CRAVER, L. F., and C. D. HAAGENSEN: A note on the occurrence of herpes zoster in Hodgkin's disease, lymphosarcoma and the leukemias. Amer. J. Cancer 16, 502—514 (1932).

CRISP, G. H.: Chickenpox and herpes zoster (Letter to Editor). Lancet 2, 311 (1940).

CRUICKSHANK, J. G., H. S. BEDSON, and D. H. WATSON: Electron microscopy in the rapid diagnosis of smallpox. Lancet 2, 527—530 (1966).

CURWEN, M. P., R. T. D. EMOND, and G. D. W. McKENDRICK: Contolled trial of A. B. O. B. in measles, chicken-pox and mumps. Brit. med. J. 1, 236—237 (1963).

DAHL, D.: Studies on the vesicles in zoster and chicken-pox. Nord. Med. 22, 1120 (1944).

DAHL, S.: Beitrag zum Studium der Epidemiologie des Herpes zoster und der Varizellen. Schweiz. med. Wschr. 76, 343—346 (1946).

DAS, P. K., and J. C. SAHA: Post-varicella polyneuritis. J. Indian med. Ass. 45, 599—601 (1965).

DAVIDSON, H. S.: Relationship between the viruses of varicella and herpes zoster. Med. Rec. (N. Y.) 139, 410—411 (1934).

DAYAN, A. D., H. G. MORGAN, H. F. HOPE-STONE, and B. J. BOUCHER: Disseminated herpes zoster in the reticuloses. Amer. J. Roentgenol. 92, 116—123 (1964).

DENNY-BROWN, D., R. D. ADAMS, and P. J. FITZGERALD: Pathologic features of herpes zoster. A note on "geniculate herpes". Arch. Neurol. Psychiat. (Chic.) 51, 216—231 (1944).

DODGE, P. R., and D. C. POSKANZER: Varicella-zoster and herpes simplex antibody responses in patients with Bell's palsy. Neurology (Minneap.) 12, 34—35 (1962).

DOHI, J., Y. OTA, F. AMANO, R. MORI, F. TAKAKI, H. YASUDA, A. SUZUKI, and T. WAKAMORI: Electron microscopic study of viral diseases. Jap. J. Derm. 71, 642—650 (1961).

DOWNIE, A. W.: Chickenpox and zoster. Brit. med. Bull. 15, 197—200 (1959).

DUEHR, P. A.: Herpes zoster as a cause of congenital cataract. Amer. J. Ophthal. 39, 157—161 (1955).

DUMBELL, K. R., and MD. NIZAMUDDIN: An agar-gel precipitation test for the laboratory diagnosis of smallpox. Lancet 1, 916—917 (1959).

DUMONT, M.: Viroses inapparentes et malformations foetales. Presse méd. 68, 1087 (1960).

DUPERRAT, B.: Le virustat en dermatologie. Sém. Hôp. Paris 39, 686—691 (1963).

EAGLSTEIN, W. H., R. KATZ, and J. A. BROWN: The effects of early corticosteroid therapy on the skin eruption and pain of herpes zoster. J. Amer. med. Ass. 211, 1681—1683 (1970).

ECKHARDT, W. F. JR., and G. W. HEBARD: Severe herpes zoster during corticosteroid therapy. Report of a severe attack in a patient with rheumatoid arthritis. Arch. intern. Med. 108, 594—598 (1961).

ECKSTEIN, A.: Klenische und experimentelle intersuchungen zur froge du varicell-encephalitis. Z. ges. Neurol. Psychiat. **149**, 176—190 (1933—1934).

EHRLICH, R. M., J. A. P. TURNER, and M. CLARKE: Neonatal varicella: a case report with isolation of the virus. J. Pediat. **53**, 139—147 (1958).

EICHENWALD, H. F., G. H. McCRACKAN, and S. J. KINDBERG: Virus infections of the newborn. Progr. med. Virol. **9**, 35—104 (1967).

EISENBUD, M.: Chickenpox with visceral involvement. Amer. J. Med. **12**, 740—746 (1952).

EISENHOFF, H. M., and M. MARCUS: Acute myositis; a complication of varicella. N. Y. J. Med. **58**, 3685—3686 (1958).

EISENKLAM, E. J.: Primary varicella pneumonia in a three-year-old girl. J. Pediat. **69**, 452—454 (1966).

ELLIOTT, F. A.: Treatment of herpes zoster with high doses of prednisone. Lancet **2**, 610—611 (1964).

EPSTEIN, E., and H. V. ALLINGTON: Treatment of herpes zoster. A. M. A. Arch. Derm. **76**, 408—412 (1957).

ESIRI, M. M., and A. H. TOMLINSON: Herpes zoster. Demonstration of virus in trigeminal nerve and ganglion by immunofluorescence and electron microscopy. J. neurol. Sci. **15**, 35—48 (1972).

EVANS, A. S., and J. L. MELNICK: Electron microscope studies of the vesicle and spinal fluids from a case of herpes zoster. Proc. Soc. exp. Biol. (N. Y.) **71**, 283—286 (1949).

EVANS, P.: An epidemic of chickenpox. Lancet **2**, 339—340 (1940).

FALLIERS, C. J., and E. F. ELLIS: Corticosteroids and varicella. Six-year experience in an asthmatic population. Arch. Dis. Child. **40**, 593—599 (1965).

FARRANT, J. L., and J. L. O'CONNOR: Elementary bodies of varicella and herpes zoster. Nature (Lond.) **163**, 260—261 (1949).

FELDMAN, G. V.: Herpes zoster neonatorum. Arch. Dis. Child. **27**, 126—127 (1952).

FERRIMAN, D. G.: Herpes zoster and chickenpox simultaneously in the same patient. Lancet **1**, 930 (1939).

FINE, R. N., H. T. WRIGHT, E. LIEBERMAN, and A. GORDON: Azathioprine and varicella. J. Amer. med. Ass. **207**, 147—148 (1969).

FINKEL, K. C.: Mortality from varicella in children receiving adrenocorticosteroids and adrenocorticotropin. Pediatrics **28**, 436—441 (1961).

FISH, S. A.: Viral diseases complicating pregnancy: practical management. Sth. med. J. (Bgham, Ala.) **58**, 1093—1098 (1965).

FITZ, R. H., and G. MEIKLEJOHN: Varicella pneumonia in adults. Amer. J. med. Sci. **233**, 489—499 (1956).

FOGH, J., and R. O. LUND: Continuous cultivation of epithelial cell strain (FL) from human amniotic membrane. Proc. Soc. exp. Biol. (N. Y.) **94**, 532—537 (1957).

FOX, M. J., E. R. KRUMBIEGEL, and J. L. TERESI: Maternal measles, mumps, and chickenpox as a cause of congenital anomalies. Lancet **1**, 746—749 (1948).

FRANDSEN, E.: Chickenpox in the cornea. Acta ophthal. (Kbh.) **28**, 113—120 (1950).

FRANK, L.: Varicella pneumonitis: report of a case with autopsy observations. Arch. Path. **50**, 450—456 (1950).

FREUD, P., G. D. ROOK, and S. GURIAN: Herpes zoster in the newborn. Report of its occurrence in a three day old infant. Amer. J. Dis. Child. **64**, 895—897 (1942).

FRY, A.: Herpes zoster and steroid therapy. Brit. med. J. **1**, 1605 (1963).

FUHLROTT: Gehäuftes Auftreten von Herpes zoster. Münch. med. Wschr. **67**, 1321 (1920).

FUNKHOUSER, W. L.: The use of serum gamma globulin antibodies to control chickenpox in a convalescent hospital for children. J. Pediat. **32**, 257—259 (1948).

GARLAND, J.: Varicella following exposure to herpes zoster. New Engl. J. Med. **228**, 336—337 (1943).

GÉDER, L., E. JENEY, and E. GÖNCZÖL: Growth of varicella virus in continuous monkey kidney and human thyroid cell cultures. Acta microbiol. Acad. Sci. hung. **11**, 361—368 (1964).

GÉDER, L., M. KOLLER, E. GÖNCZÖL, E. JENEY, and I. GÖNCZÖL: Isolation of herpes zoster virus strains. Acta microbiol. Acad. Sci. hung. **10**, 155—161 (1963).

GÉDER, L., L. VÁCZI, and M. KOLLER: Persistent varicella and herpes simplex infection of a continuous monkey kidney cell culture. Acta virol. **9**, 431—436 (1965).

GEY, G. O., W. D. COFFMAN, and M. T. KUBICEK: Tissue culture studies of the proliferative capacity of cervical carcinoma and normal epithelium. Cancer Res. **12**, 264 (1952).

GIBBS, R. C., E. SHAPIRO, H. CASSIDY, and P. A. BRUNELL: Possible mechanisms for maintaining immunity to varicella-zoster virus. Clinical observations. Amer. J. Dis. Child. **120**, 456—457 (1970).

GIRSH, L. S., M. YU, J. JONES, and F. A. SCHULANER: A study of the risk of mortality of varicella in patients with bronchial asthma or other allergic disease receiving corticosteroid therapy. Ann. Allergy **24**, 690—693 (1966).

GOLD, E.: Characteristics of herpes zoster and varicella viruses propagated *in vitro*. J. Immunol. **95**, 683—691 (1965).

GOLD, E.: Serologic and virus isolation studies of patients with varicella or herpes zoster infection. New Engl. J. Med. **274**, 181—185 (1966).

GOLD, E., and G. GODEK: Complement fixation studies with a varicella-zoster antigen. J. Immunol. **95**, 692—695 (1965).

GOLD E., and F. C. ROBBINS: Isolation of herpes zoster virus from spinal fluid of a patient. Virology **6**, 293—295 (1958).

GOLEMBA, P. I.: Epidemiology of herpes zoster. Pediatriya (Moskva) **41**, 59 (1958).

GOOD, R. A., R. L. VERNIER and R. T. SMITH: Serious untoward reactions to therapy with cortisone and adrenocorticotropin in pediatric practice. Pediatrics **19**, 95—118 (1957).

GOODPASTURE, E. W., and K. ANDERSON: Infection of human skin, grafted on the chorioallantois of chick embryos, with the virus of herpes zoster. Amer. J. Path. **20**, 447—455 (1944).

GORDON, J. E.: Chickenpox: an epidemiological review. Amer. J. med. Sci. **244**, 362—389 (1962).

GORDON, J. E., and F. M. MEADER: The period of infectivity and serum prevention of chickenpox. J. Amer. med. Ass. **93**, 2013—2015 (1929).

GORDON, I. R. S., and J. F. TUCKER: Lesions of the central nervous system in herpes zoster. J. Neurol. Neurosurg. Psychiat. **8**, 40—46 (1945).

G. P. clinical trials: A trial of "virugon" in herpes zoster. Practitioner **195**, 235—237 (1965).

GRAHAM-LITTLE, E.: Recurrent idiopathic herpes zoster. Brit. med. J. **1**, 498 (1937).

GRANT, B. D., and C. R. ROWE: Motor paralysis of the extremities in herpes zoster. J. Bone Joint Surg. **43 A**, 885—896 (1961).

GREENBERG, J.: Herpes zoster with motor involvement. J. Amer. med. Ass. **212**, 322 (1970).

GREENBERG, M.: Gamma globulin in pediatrics. Med. Clin. N. Amer. **31**, 602—608 (1947).

GREENE, D., L. H. BARENBERG, and B. GREENBERG: Effect of radiation of the air in a ward on the incidence of infections of the respiratory tract, with a note on varicella. Amer. J. Dis. Child. **61**, 273—275 (1941).

GREENTHAL, R. M.: The prophylaxis of varicella with vesicle fluid. Amer. J. Dis. Child. **31**, 851—855 (1926).

GRIFFIN, W. P., and C. W. A. SEARLE: Ocular manifestations of varicella. Lancet **2**, 168—169 (1953).

GRIPENBERG, U.: Chromosome studies in some virus infections. Hereditas **54**, 1—18 (1965).

GRIVEL, M.-L.: Récidives de varicelle chez deux asthmatiques? Ann. Pédiat. **157**, 253—254 (1941).

GROS, H.: Die Behandlung des Herpes zoster mit Humanglobulin. Dtsch. med. Wschr. **77**, 1074—1076 (1952).

GROUCHY, J. DE, V. TUDELA et J. FEINGOLD: Études cytogénétiques "in vivo" et "in vitro" après infections virales et après vaccination anti-amarile. Path. et Biol. (Paris) 15, 879—885 (1967).

GULÁCSY, Z.: Aktive Schutzimpfung gegen Varizellen. Arch. Kinderheilk. 100, 75—80 (1933).

GUNALP, A.: Growth and cytopathic effect of rubella virus in a line of green monkey kidney cells. Proc. Soc. exp. Biol. (N. Y.) 118, 85—90 (1965).

GUNN, W.: Convalescent serum in prophylaxis of measles, chickenpox and mumps with observations on variations in the Wassermann reaction. Brit. med. J. 1, 183—185 (1932).

GURVICH, E. B.: On the isolation and cultivation of chickenpox and herpes zoster viruses in tissue culture. Vop. Virus. 7, 706—712 (1962).

HACKEL, D. B.: Myocarditis in association with varicella. Amer. J. Path. 29, 369—379 (1953).

HAGGERTY, R. J., and R. C. ELEY: Varicella and cortisone. Pediatrics 18, 160—162 (1956).

HALL, P.: Korsakov's syndrome following herpes-zoster encephalitis. Lancet 1, 752 (1963).

HALPERN, S. L., and A. H. COVNER: Motor manifestations of herpes zoster. Arch. intern. Med. 84, 907—916 (1949).

HAMPARIAN, V. V., M. R. HILLEMAN, and A. KETLER: Contributions to characterization and classification of animal viruses. Proc. Soc. exp. Biol. (N. Y.) 112, 1040—1050 (1963).

HARDY, J. B.: Viral infection in pregnancy: A review. Amer. J. Obstet. Gynec. 93, 1052—1956 (1965).

HARNDEN, D. G.: Cytogenetic studies on patients with virus infections and subjects vaccinated against yellow fever. Amer. J. hum. Genet. 16, 204—213 (1964).

HARPER, J. R., R. D. MARSHALL, and M. S. PARKINSON: Intermittent positive-pressure ventilation in chicken-pox pneumonitis. Brit. med. J. 2, 637—638 (1969).

HARRIES, E. H. R., M. MITMAN, and I. TAYLOR: "Clinical Practice in Infectious Diseases". 4th edit. pp. 341—352, Edinburgh: E. and S. Livingstone Ltd. 1951.

HASLUND, A.: Festschrift Moriz Kaposi, pp. 169—182. Zona als Infektionskrankheit. Arch. Derm. Syph. (Berl.) Ergänzungsbd. (1900).

HASSKÓ, A., L. VAMOS und M. THOROCZKAY: Über die Komplementbindung der Sera von Herpes und von Varizellen. Z. Immunforsch. 93, 80—86 (1938).

HAYES, J. A., T. E. BEEN, E. J. VALENTINE, and G. BRAS: A case of fatal dissemination of varicella. J. Path. Bact. 90, 328—333 (1965).

HAYFLICK, L., and P. S. MOORHEAD: The serial cultivation of human diploid cell strains. Exp. Cell Res. 25, 585—621 (1961).

HEAD, H., and A. W. CAMPBELL: The pathology of herpes zoster and its bearing on sensory localisation. Brain 23, 353—523 (1900).

HELLGREN, L., and K. HERSLE: A statistical and clinical study of herpes zoster. Geront. clin. (Basel) 8, 70—76 (1966).

HERRMANN, E. C.: Experiences in laboratory diagnosis of herpes simplex, varicella-zoster, and vaccinia virus infections in routine medical practice. Mayo Clin. Proc. 42, 744—753 (1967).

HERZBERG, K., A. K. KLEINSCHMIDT, D. LANG, K. REUSS und R. DAHN: Über die Struktur des Zoster-Virus und eine weitere Darstellungsmöglichkeit seiner Capsomeren. Zbl. Bakt. I. Abt. Orig. 189, 1—13 (1963 a).

HERZBERG, K., A. K. KLEINSCHMIDT, D. LANG, K. REUSS und R. DAHN: Vergleichende Virusdarstellung mit Phosphorwolframsäure. Zbl. Bact. I. Abt. Orig. 188, 440—443 (1963 b).

HERZBERG, K., D. LANG, K. REUSS und R. DAHN: Über das Verhalten der Filamente des Kanarienpocken-Virus und der Capsomeren des Varizellen-Zostervirus gegenüber Lösemitteln und Fermenten. Zbl. Bact. I. Abt. Orig. 195, 133—143 (1964).

HESS, A. F., and L. J. UNGER: A protective therapy for varicella, and a consideration of its pathogenesis. Amer. J. Dis. Child. 16, 34—38 (1918).

HEUSCHELE, W. P.: Varicella (chicken pox) in three young anthropoid apes. J. Amer. vet. med. Ass. **136**, 256—257 (1960).

HILL, A. B., R. DOLL, T. McL. GALLOWAY, and J. P. W. HUGHES: Virus diseases in pregnancy and congenital defects. Brit. J. prev. soc. Med. **12**, 1—7 (1958).

HOLBROOK, A. A.: The coincidence of chickenpox and lymphatic leukemia. New Engl. J. Med. **216**, 598—603 (1937).

HOPE-SIMPSON, R. E.: The nature of herpes zoster. Practitioner **193**, 217—219 (1964).

HOPE-SIMPSON, R. E.: The nature of herpes zoster: a long-term study and a new hypothesis. Proc. roy. Soc. Med. **58**, 9—20 (1965).

HOPE-SIMPSON, R. E.: Herpes zoster in the elderly. Geriatrics **22**, 151—159 (1967).

HOPPS, H. E., B. C. BERNHEIM, A. NISALAK, J. HIN TJIO, and J. E. SMADEL: Biologic characteristics of a continuous kidney cell line derived from the African green monkey. J. Immunol. **91**, 416—424 (1963).

HORTON, S. H. JR.: Herpes zoster following exposure to varicella: treatment of herpes zoster with coxpox vaccine. U. S. Nav. med. Bull. **48**, 742—749 (1948).

HUBBARD, T. W.: Varicella occurring in an infant twenty-four hours after birth. Brit. med. J. **1**, 822 (1878).

HUGHES, R. P., and L. M. SMITH: Varicella occurring twice in one patient during a single epidemic. Arch. Derm. Syph. **40**, 433 (1939).

HUNT, J. R.: On herpetic inflammations of the geniculate ganglion. A new syndrome and its complications. J. nerv. ment. Dis. **34**, 73—96 (1907).

HUTTON, P. W.: Bilateral zoster and zoster varicellosus. Lancet **2**, 302—303 (1935).

HYATT, H. W.: Neonatal varicella. Report of a case in a 5-day-old infant and review of the literature. J. nat. med. Ass. (N. Y.) **59**, 32—34 (1967).

IOULEV, V. I., L. M. BOICHUK, A. T. KUZMICHERA, and A. A. SMORODINTSEV: Reactogenic and immunogenic properties of an attenuated strain of varicella virus. Vop. Virus. **14**, 249—250 (1969).

IRIARTE, P. V., A. TANGCO, K. H. JAGASIA, R. DIESCHE, and W. G. THURMAN: Effect of gamma globulin on modification of chickenpox in children with malignant disease. Cancer **18**, 112—116 (1965).

IRONS, J. V., S. W. BOHLS, E. B. M. COOK, and J. N. MURPHY: The chick membrane as a differential culture medium with suspected cases of smallpox and varicella. Amer. J. Hyg. **33** B, 50—55 (1941).

JOHNSON, H. N.: Visceral lesions associated with varicella. Arch. Path. **30**, 292—307 (1940).

JOHNSON, R. T.: Spread of herpes-zoster virus. New Engl. J. Med. **278**, 743 (1968).

JOHNSON, R. T., and C. A. MIMS: Pathogenesis of viral infections of the nervous system. New Engl. J. Med. **278**, 23—30; 84—92 (1968).

JUEL-JENSEN, B. E.: Results of the treatment of zoster with idoxuridine in dimethyl-sulphoxide. Ann. N. Y. Acad. Sci. **173**, 74—82 (1970).

JUEL-JENSEN, B. E.: The natural history of shingles: events associated with reactivation of varicella-zoster virus. J. roy. Coll. gen. Pract. **20**, 323—327 (1970).

KALB, O.: Über angeborene multiple, symmetrisch gruppierte Narbenbildungen im Gesicht. Zbl. Gynäk. **33**, 929—931 (1909).

KAPLAN, L., and J. B. TULLY: Visceral "viral" dissemination in a patient with bronchogenic carcinoma. Arch. Path. **56**, 312—322 (1953).

KAPSENBERG, J. G.: Possible antigenic relationship between varicella-zoster virus and herpes simplex virus. Arch. ges. Virusforsch. **15**, 67—73 (1964).

KASS, E. H., R. R. AYCOCK, and M. FINLAND: Clinical evaluation of aureomycin and chloramphenicol in herpes zoster. New Engl. J. Med. **246**, 167—172 (1952).

KATAYAMA, K.: Klinisch-statistische Beobachtungen über Herpes zoster. Jap. J. Derm. Urol. **43**, 145—146 (1938).

KEIDAN, S. E., and D. MAINWARING: Association of herpes zoster with leukaemia and lymphoma in children. Clin. Pediat. **4**, 13—17 (1965).

KIBRICK, S., and A. S. KATZ: Topical idoxuridine in recurrent herpes simplex. With a note on its effect on early varicella. Ann. N. Y. Acad. Sci. **173**, 83—89 (1970).

KIMURA, A., TOSAKA, K., and T. NAKAO: An electron microscopic study of varicella skin lesions. Arch. ges. Virusforsch. **36**, 1—12 (1972).

KIN, O.: Study of zostervirus. I. Report: on animal inoculation of Herpes zoster virus. Jap. J. Derm. Urol. **46**, 133—134 (1939).

KIN O.: Studien über Zostervirus. Jap. J. Derm. Urol. **47**, 39 (1940).

KISSLING, R. E., H. L. CASEY, and E. L. PALMER: Production of specific varicella antiserum. Appl. Microbiol. **16**, 160—162 (1968).

KLING, C. A.: Technik der Schutzimpfung gegen Varicella. Berl. klin. Wschr. **52**, 13—15 (1915).

KNIGHT, V., W. F. FLEET, and D. J. LANG: Inhibition of measles rash by chickenpox. J. Amer. med. Ass. **188**, 690—691 (1964).

KNYVETT, A. F.: The pulmonary lesions of chickenpox. Quart. J. Med. **35**, 313—323 (1966).

KOLLER, M., E. GÖNCZÖL, and I. VÁCZI: Study of the multiplication of varicella-zoster virus by the fluorescent antibody test. Acta microbiol. Acad. Sci. hung. **10**, 183—188 (1963).

KÖRNER, O.: Über den Herpes zoster oticus. (Herpes an der Ohrmuschel mit Lähmung des Nervus acusticus und des Nervus facialis.) Münch. med. Wschr. **1**, 6—7 (1904).

KRECH, U., and M. JUNG: Antigenic relationship between human cytomegalovirus, herpes simplex, and varicella-zoster virus studied by complement-fixation. Arch. ges. Virusforsch. **33**, 288—295 (1971).

KRUGMAN, S.: Varicella and herpes virus infections. Pediat. Clin. N. Amer. **7**, 881—902 (1960).

KRUMHOLZ, S., and J. A. LUHAN: Encephalitis associated with herpes zoster. Report of a case. Arch. Neurol. Psychiat. **53**, 59—67 (1945).

KUNDRATITZ, K.: Über die Ätiologie des Zoster und über seine Beziehungen zu Varizellen. Wien. klin. Wschr. **38**, 502—503 (1925).

LAFORET, E. G., and C. L. LYNCH: Multiple congenital defects following maternal varicella. Report of a case. New Engl. J. Med. **236**, 534—537 (1947).

LANGE, C. DE: Herpes zoster varicellosa Bokay und Varicellen. Klin. Wschr. **2**, 879—880 (1923).

LAUDA, E., und E. SILBERSTERN: Zur Frage der serologischen Beziehungen zwischen Zoster und Varicellen. Klin. Wschr. **4**, 1871—1872 (1925).

LEA, A. W. JR., and W. B. TAYLOR: γ-globulin in the treatment of herpes zoster. Tex. J. Med. **54**, 594—596 (1958).

LEAK, W. N.: Recurrent chickenpox (Letter to Editor). Lancet **2**, 375 (1940).

LE FEUVRE, W. P.: A plea for the recognition of a common origin for shingles and chickenpox. Brit. J. Derm. **29**, 253—262 (1917).

LEONARD, L. L., N. J. SCHMIDT, and E. H. LENNETTE: Demonstration of viral antibody activity in two immunoglobulin G subclasses in patients with varicella-zoster virus infection. J. Immunol. **104**, 23—27 (1970).

LEVADITI, C.: "L'Herpès et le Zona", pp. 28—35. Paris: Masson et Cie., 1926.

LEWIS, G. W.: Zoster sine herpete. Brit. med. J. **2**, 418—421 (1958).

LEWIS, J. M., L. H. BARENBERG, and G. GROSSMAN: Convalescent serum in the prevention of chickenpox. Amer. J. Dis. Child. **53**, 750—753 (1937).

LIEBHABER, H., J. T. RIORDAN, and D. M. HORSTMANN: Replication of rubella virus in a continuous line of African green monkey cells (Vero). Proc. Soc. exp. Biol. (N. Y.) **125**, 636—643 (1967).

LIPSCHÜTZ, B.: Untersuchungen über die Ätiologie der Krankheiten der Herpesgruppe (Herpes zoster, Herpes genitalis, Herpes febrilis). Arch. Derm. Syph. (Berl.) **136**, 428—482 (1921).

LOEBL, W. Y., and C. E. D. TAYLOR: Treatment of varicella. Lancet **1**, 1037 (1966).

LOMER: Herpes zooster bei einem 4 Tage alten Kinde. Zbl. Gynäk. **13**, 778—779 (1889).

LORANT, A.: Effect of surgical scar on herpes zoster. New Engl. J. Med. **278**, 397 (1968).

LOW, R. C.: Herpes zoster: its cause, and association with varicella. Brit. med. J. **1**, 91—92 (1919).

LUCCHESI, P. F., A. C. LABOCCETTA, and A. R. PEALE: Varicella neonatorum. Amer. J. Dis. Child. **73**, 44—54 (1947).

LUTZNER, M. A.: Fine structure of the zoster virus in human skin. J. Ultrastruct. Res. **7**, 409—417 (1962).

LUTZNER, M. A.: Molluscum contagiosum, verruca and zoster viruses. Arch. Derm. **87**, 436—444 (1963).

LUX, S. E., R. B. JOHNSTON, C. S. AUGUST, B. SAY, V. B. PENCHASZADEH, F. S. ROSEN, and V. A. McKUSICK: Chronic neutropenia and abnormal cellular immunity in cartilage-hair hypoplasia. New Engl. J. Med., **282**, 231—236 (1970).

MACKAY, J. B., and P. CAIRNEY: Pulmonary calcification following varicella. N. Z. med. J. **59**, 453—457 (1960).

MACRAE, A. D., A. M. FIELD, J. R. McDONALD, E. V. MEURISSE, and A. A. PORTER: Laboratory differential diagnosis of vesicular skin rashes. Lancet **2**, 313—316 (1969).

MAGNUSSON, J. H.: Studien über Zoster. Impfversuche an Affen mit Material von Zosterfällen. Acta paediat. (Uppsala) **28**, 323—343 (1941).

MALANINA, G. I.: Herpes zoster as a disease simulating "acute abdomen". Khirurgiya (Mosk.) **41**, 134—135 (1965).

MANDELBAUM, J., and B. H. TERK: Pericarditis in association with chickenpox. J. Amer. med. Ass. **170**, 191—194 (1959).

MANSON, M. M., W. P. D. LOGAN, and R. M. LOY: Rubella and other virus infections during pregnancy. Ministry of Health Reports on Public Health and Medical Subjects — No. 101. Her Majesty's Stationery Office (1960).

MARAN, J. I., S. S. LAWSON, A. F. HILE, and J. S. BALL: Treatment of herpes simplex and zoster with terramycin. J. Coll. gen. Practit. **13**, 110—114 (1967).

MARETIć, Z., and M. P. M. COORAY: Comparisons between chickenpox in a tropical and a European country. J. trop. Med. Hyg. **66**, 311—315 (1963).

MARTOS, L. M., D. V. ABLASHI, R. V. GILDEN, R. F. SIGÜENZA, and B. HAMPAR: Preparation of immune rabbit sera with neutralizing activity against human cytomegalovirus and varicella-zoster virus. J. gen. Virol. **7**, 169—171 (1970).

MASSARELLI, J. J.: Spread of herpes-zoster virus. New Engl. J. Med., **278**, 743 (1968).

MASSIMO, L., M. G. VIANELLO, F. DAGNA-BRICARELLI, and G. TORTOROLO: Fetopathy caused by varicella and acquired chromosomal aberrations. Presentation of a case. G. Mal. infett. **17**, 849—853 (1965).

McCALLUM, D. I.: Herpes zoster varicellosus. Brit. med. J. **1**, 520—523 (1952).

McCALLUM, D. I.: Herpes zoster treated with I. D. U. Brit. med. J. **1**, 1288—1289 (1963).

McCALLUM, D. I., E. N. M. JOHNSTON, and B. H. RAJU: 5-iodo-2'-deoxyuridine in the treatment of herpes zoster. Brit. J. Derm. **76**, 459—462 (1964).

McCORMICK, W. F., R. L. RODNITZKY, S. S. SCHOCHET, and A. P. McKEE: Varicella-zoster encephalomyelitis. A morphologic and virologic study. Arch. Neurol. **21**, 559—570 (1969).

McDONAGH, T. J.: Passive immunization with gamma globulin. J. occup. Med. **8**, 567—572 (1966).

McEWEN, E. L.: The association of herpes zoster and varicella. Arch. Derm. Syph. (Chic.) **2**, 205—214 (1920).

McGREGOR, R. M.: Herpes zoster, chickenpox, and cancer in general practice. Brit. med. J. **1**, 84—87 (1957).

McKHANN, C. F., A. STEEGER, and A. P. LONG: Hospital infections. I. A survey of the problem. Amer. J. Dis. Child. **55**, 579—599 (1938).

McMATH, W. F. T., and K. K. HUSSAIN: Investigation of ultraviolet radiation in the control of chickenpox cross-infection. Brit. J. clin. Pract. **14**, 19—21 (1960).

Medical Research Council special report series No. 227. Epidemics in schools. An analysis of the data collected during the first five years of a statistical inquiry by the School Epidemics Committee, pp. 181—184 (1938).

MELNICK, J. L., M. MIDULLA, I. WIMBERLY, J. G. BARRERA-ORO, and B. M. LEVY: A new member of the herpes-virus group isolated from South American marmosets. J. Immunol. **92**, 596—601 (1964).

MENUT, G., J. C. DIEU et F. ADENIS-LAMARRE: Les echecs d'une chimiothérapie anti-virale (ABOB) au cours d'une épidémie de varicelle. Arch. franç. Pédiat. **21**, 859—869 (1964).

MERIGAN, T. C., D. WADDELL, M. GROSSMAN, J. H. RITCHIE, and G. MO: Modified skin lesions during concurrent varicella and measles infections. J. Amer. med. Ass. **204**, 333—335 (1968).

MERSELIS, J. G., D. KAYE, and E. W. HOOK: Disseminated herpes zoster. A report of 17 cases. Arch. intern. Med. **113**, 679—686 (1964).

MEURISSE, E. V.: Laboratory studies on the varicella-zoster virus. J. med. Microbiol. **2**, 317—325 (1969).

MILLER, L. H., and P. A. BRUNELL: Zoster, reinfection or activation of latent virus? Observations on the antibody response. Amer. J. Med. **49**, 480—483 (1970).

MILLOUS, M.: Une épidémie de varicelle maligne au Cameroun. Bull. Acad. Méd. (Paris) **115**, 840—843 (1936).

MITCHELL, A. G., and E. G. FLETCHER: Studies on varicella. J. Amer. med. Ass. **89**, 279—280 (1927).

MONTALDO, G., W. TANGHERONI e A. FALORNI: Reperti al microscopio elettronico di ultrastrutture e di virus nelle vescicole di varicella. Arch. De Vecchi Anat. pat. **48**, 1—18 (1966).

MONTGOMERY, D. W.: Herpes zoster as a primary ascending neuritis. Arch. Derm. Syph. (Chic.) **4**, 812—817 (1921).

MORTON, O.: Herpes zoster. Curr. Med. Drugs **8**, 19—31 (1968).

MOSCOVITZ, H. L.: Generalized herpes zoster initiating a minor epidemic of chickenpox J. Mt. Sinai Hosp. **22**, 79—90 (1955).

MOZHAEV, V. I.: Herpes zoster as a disease simulating acute abdomen. Klin. Med. (Moskva) **42**, 115—116 (1964).

MULLER, S. A.: Association of zoster and malignant disorders in children. Arch. Derm. **96**, 657—664 (1967).

NAGLER, F. P. O., and G. RAKE: The use of the electron microscope in diagnosis of variola, vaccinia and varicella. J. Bact. **55**, 45—51 (1948).

NELSON, A. M., and J. W. St. GEME, JR.: On the respiratory spread of varicella-zoster virus. Pediatrics **37**, 1007—1009 (1966).

NETTER, A.: Discussion on varicella and zoster. Bull. Soc. méd. Hôp., Paris **52**, 1014—1020 (1928).

NETTER, A., et A., URBAIN: Zonas varicelleux. Anticorps varicelleux dans le sérum de sujets atteints de zona. Anticorps zostériens et anticorps varicelleux dans le sérum de sujets atteints de varicelle. C. R. Soc. Biol. (Paris) **90**, 189—191 (1924 a).

NETTER, A., et A., URBAIN: Nouvelles recherches sur la déviation du complément dans le zona. L'antigène du zona n'exerce aucune action sur le sérum des sujets atteints d'herpès. C. R. Soc. Biol. (Paris) **90**, 461—464 (1924 b).

NETTER, A., et A., URBAIN: Les relations du zona et de la varicelle. Etude sérologique de 100 cas de zona. C. R. Soc. Biol. (Paris) **94**, 98—102 (1926).

NETTER, A., A. URBAIN et WEISSMANN-NETTER: Antigènes et anticorps dans le zona. C. R. Soc. Biol. (Paris) **90**, 75—76 (1924).

NETTER, R.: Études sur le virus de la varicelle. Path. et Biol. (Paris) **12**, 467—471 (1964).

NETTER, R., et A.-M. SIBILAT: Application de l'immune-électrophorèse croisée au diagnostic différentiel rapide entre poxvirus et virus varicello-zonateux. Bull. Wld Hlth Org. **39**, 940—941 (1968).

NICHOLS, W. W.: Experiences with chickenpox in patients with hematologic disease receiving cortisone. Amer. J. Dis. Child. **94**, 219—223 (1957).

NICOLAU, S., et L. KOPIOWSKA: La morphologie de l'inframicrobe herpétique dans le tissue des animaux infectés expérimentalement et le mechanisme de la formation des inclusions qu'il engendre dans les cellules. Ann. Inst. Pasteur **60**, 401—431 (1938).

NII, S., and Y. MAEDA: Studies of Herpes zoster in vitro. 1. Isolation of two variants. Biken J. **12**, 219—230 (1969).

NII, S., and Y. MAEDA: Studies of Herpes zoster virus in vitro. 2. An auto-radiographic study of intra-nuclear inclusions. Biken J. **13**, 133—144 (1970).

NIVEN, J. S. F.: Induced fluorescent microscopy of virus infected cells. 5th International Poliomyelitis Conference, Copenhagen, Denmark, July 26—28, 1960. pp. 53—62. Philadelphia: Lippincott, 1961.

OPPENHEIMER, E. H.: Congenital chickenpox with disseminated visceral lesions. Johns Hopk. Hosp. Bull. **74**, 240—250 (1944).

OUCHTERLONY, Ö.: In vitro method for testing the toxin-producing capacity of diphtheria bacteria. Acta path. microbiol. scand. **25**, 186—191 (1948).

PARK, W. H.: A practical method for differentiating between variola and varicella by means of the inoculation of monkeys. Trans. Ass. Amer. Phycns **17**, 217—221 (1902).

PASCHEN, E.: Vergleichende Untersuchungen von Varizellen, Variola, Scharlach, Masern und Röteln. Dtsch. med. Wschr. **43**, 746—747 (1917).

PASCHEN, E.: In discussion. Hyg. Rdsch. **29**, 313—314 (1919).

PASCHEN, E.: 1. Weitere Mitteilungen über Vakzineviruszüchtung in der Gewebekultur. 2. Elementarkörperchen im Bläscheninhalt bei Herpes Zoster und Varizellen. Zbl. Bakt. I. Abt. Orig. **130**, 190—193 (1933).

PATENKO, V. M.: The interaction of chickenpox virus with cells of the chick embryo chorio-allantois. Veterinariya **43**, 34—37 (1966).

PEARSON, H. E.: Parturition varicella-zoster. Obstet. and Gynec. **23**, 21—27 (1964).

PEITERSEN, E., and A. E. CAUNT: The incidence of herpes zoster antibodies in patients with peripheral facial palsy. J. Laryng. **84**, 65—70 (1970).

PERIER, O., J. J. VANDERHAEGHEN, and L. FRANKEN: Clinical and anatomical study of 2 cases of zosterial encephalitis. Review and discussion of the literature. Acta neurol. belg. **66**, 53—75 (1966).

PESTEL, M.: Le zona. Presse méd. **69**, 347—348 (1961).

PETERSON, P. H., and S. A. B. BLACK: Varicella herpetiformis. Brit. med. J. **1**, 762 (1946).

PICKARD, R. E.: Varicella pneumonia in pregnancy. Amer. J. Obstet. Gynec. **101**, 504—508 (1968).

PICKLES, W. N.: "Epidemiology in Country Practice". 1st ed., pp. 45—50, Bristol: Wright, 1939.

PINKEL, D.: Chickenpox and leukemia. J. Pediat. **58**, 729—737 (1961).

PLUMMER, G.: Comparative virology of the herpes group. Progr. med. Virol. **9**, 302—340 (1967).

PRIDHAM, F. C.: Chicken-pox during intrauterine life. Brit. med. J. **1**, 1054 (1913).

RADO, J. P., J. TAKO, L. GÉDER, and E. JENEY: Herpes zoster house epidemic in steroid-treated patients. A clinical and viral study. Arch. intern. Med. (Chic.) **116**, 329—335 (1965).

RAINE, D. N.: Varicella infection contracted in utero: sex incidence and incubation period. Amer. J. Obstet. Gynec. **94**, 1144—1145 (1966).

RAKE, G., H. BLANK, L. L. CORIELL, F. P. O. NAGLER, and T. F. M. SCOTT: The relationship of varicella and herpes zoster: electron microscopic study. J. Bact. **56**, 293—303 (1948).

RAMOND, L., et R. LEBEL: L'adénite primitive du zona. Bull. Soc. méd. Hôp. Paris **44**, 1157—1162 (1920).

RAPP, F.: Inhibition by metabolic analogues of plaque formation by herpes zoster and herpes simplex viruses. J. Immunol. **93**, 643—648 (1964).

RAPP, F., and M. BENYESH-MELNICK: Plaque assay for measurement of cells infected with zoster virus. Science **141**, 433—434 (1963).

RAPP, F., and D. VANDERSLICE: Spread of zoster virus in human embryonic lung cells and the inhibitory effect of iododeoxyuridine. Virology **22**, 321—330 (1964).

RAWLS, W. E., R. A. COHEN, and E. C. HERRMANN, JR.: Inhibition of varicella virus by 5-iodo-2'-deoxyuridine. Proc. Soc. exp. Biol. (N. Y.) **115**, 123—127 (1964).

RAWLS, W. E., and E. C. HERRMANN, JR.: Human placenta as a source of fibroblasts for viral studies. Amer. J. Hyg. **80**, 266—274 (1964).

READETT, M. D., and C. L. McGIBBON: Neonatal varicella. Lancet **1**, 644—645 (1961).

REAGAN, R. L., W. C. DAY, S. MOORE, and A. L. BRUECKNER: Electron microscopic studies of the virus of varicella (chicken pox) from monkey serum. Tex. Rep. Biol. Med. **11**, 74—78 (1953).

REED, D., J. A. BRODY, G. SPERRY, and J. SEVER: Methisazone for prophylaxis against chickenpox. J. Amer. med. Ass. **195**, 586—588 (1966).

REICH, J. S., and A. BAUMAL: Herpes zoster and varicella occurring in siblings following contact with chickenpox. J. Mt. Sinai Hosp. **28**, 473—474 (1961).

RHYS-LEWIS, R. D. S.: Radiotherapy in herpes zoster. Lancet **2**, 102—104 (1965).

RIFKIND, D.: The activation of varicella-zoster virus infections by immunosuppressive therapy. J. Lab. clin. Med. **68**, 463—474 (1966).

RIGDON, R. H., S. A. SHOJAII, and E. P. GARBER: Fatal chickenpox: a review of the literature and a report of a case. Amer. Practit. **13**, 292—302 (1962).

RIVERS, T. M.: Nuclear inclusions in the testicles of monkeys injected with the tissue of human varicella lesions. J. exp. Med. **43**, 275—287 (1926).

RIVERS, T. M.: Varicella in monkeys. Nuclear inclusions produced by varicella virus in the testicles of monkeys. J. exp. Med. **45**, 961—968 (1927).

RIVERS, T. M., and L. A. ELDRIDGE: Relation of varicella to herpes zoster. I. Statistical observations. II. Clinical and experimental observations. J. exp. Med. **49**, 899—917 (1929).

RIVERS, T. M., and W. S. TILLET: Studies on varicella. The susceptibility of rabbits to the virus of varicella. J. exp. Med. **38**, 673—690 (1923).

RIVERS, T. M., and W. S. TILLET: Further observations on the phenomena encountered in attempting to transmit varicella to rabbits. J. exp. Med. **39**, 777—802 (1924 a).

RIVERS, T. M., and W. S. TILLET: The lesions in rabbits experimentally infected by a virus encountered in the attempted transmission of varicella. J. exp. Med. **40**, 281—287 (1924 b).

RODARTE, J. G., and B. H. WILLIAMS: Treatment of herpes zoster and chickenpox with immune globulin. Arch. Derm. **73**, 553—555 (1956).

RODNAN, G. P., and G. W. RAKE: Disseminated herpes zoster complicating chronic lymphatic leukemia. New Engl. J. Med. **254**, 472—474 (1956).

ROLLESTON, J. D.: Varicella in old age. Brit. med. J. **2**, 1007—1008 (1932).

ROSANOFF, E. I.: Observations on the growth of varicella virus and adenovirus on human diploid cell strains. International Association of Microbiological Societies. Permanent section on Microbiological Standardization. Symposium: The characterization and uses of human diploid cell strains. Yugoslavia (1963).

ROSANOFF, E. I., and C. P. HEGARTY: Preservation of tissue cultured varicella virus in the frozen state. Virology **22**, 284 (1964).

ROSCHLAU, G.: Generalized fatal varicella during high dosage corticosteroid therapy. Report of 2 cases. Münch. med. Wschr. **109**, 1889—1892 (1967).

ROSS, A. H.: Modification of chickenpox in family contacts by administration of gamma globulin. New Engl. J. Med. **267**, 369—376 (1962).

ROSS, C. A. C., J. A. R. LENMAN, and I. D. MELVILLE: Virus antibody levels in multiple sclerosis. Brit. med. J. **2**, 512—513 (1969).

ROSS, C. A. C., J. A. R. LENMAN, and C. RUTTER: Infective agents and multiple sclerosis. Brit. med. J. **1**, 226—229 (1965 a).

ROSS, C. A. C., J. H. SUBAK-SHARPE, and P. FERRY: Antigenic relationship of varicella-zoster and herpes simplex. Lancet **2**, 708—711 (1965 b).

ROTEM, C. E.: Complications of chickenpox. Brit. med. J. **1**, 944—947 (1961).

RUBIN, D., and R. D. FUSFELD: Muscle paralysis in herpes zoster. Calif. Med. **103**, 261—266 (1965).

RUSKA, H.: Über das Virus der Varizellen und des Zoster. Klin. Wschr. **22**, 703—704 (1943 a).

RUSKA, H.: Ziele und Erfolge der Uebermikroskopie in der medizinischen Forschung. Scientia (Milano) **37**, 16 (1943 b).

RUSTI, J.: Propagation de la rougeole, de la varicelle et des oreillons, enrayée par une nouvelle méthode de prophylaxie dans un sanatorium pour enfants de deux cents lits. Rev. Immunol. **21**, 393—396 (1957).

RUZICSKA, P.: Establishment of cell strains from primary monkey kidney cell cultures. Acta. morph. Acad. Sci. hung. 12, 275—287 (1964).

SALMON, P.: Diagnostic expérimental de la variole et de la varicelle. C. R. Soc. Biol. (Paris) 58, 262—263 (1905).

SCHAEFFER, M., and J. A. TOOMEY: Failure of gamma globulin to prevent varicella. J. Pediat. 33, 749—752 (1948).

SCHAFFER, A. J.: Diseases of the Newborn. 2nd Edit. London: Saunders, 1965.

SCHAPP, G. J. P., and J. HUISMAN: Simultaneous rise in complement-fixing antibodies against herpesvirus hominis and varicella-zoster virus in patients with chickenpox and shingles. Arch. ges. Virusforsch. 25, 52—57 (1968).

SCHERSTEN, B.: Treatment of herpes zoster with N'-N'-anhydrobis (β-oxyethyl) biguanide HCL (ABOB). Svenska Läh.-Tidn. 57, 3563—3566 (1959).

SCHIFF, C. I., and W. R. BRAIN: Acute meningo-encephalitis associated with herpes zoster. A fatal case. Lancet 2, 70—71 (1930).

SCHMIDT, N. J., H. H. HO, and E. H. LENNETTE: Comparative sensitivity of human fetal diploid kidney cell strains and monkey kidney cell cultures for isolation of certain human viruses. Amer. J. clin. Path. 43, 297—301 (1965 a).

SCHMIDT, N. J., E. H. LENNETTE, and R. L. MAGOFFIN: Immunological relationship between herpes simplex and varicella-zoster viruses demonstrated by complement-fixation, neutralization and fluorescent antibody tests. J. gen. Virol. 4, 321—328 (1969).

SCHMIDT, N. J., E. H. LENNETTE, C. W. SHON, and T. T. SHINOMOTO: A complement-fixing antigen for varicella-zoster derived from infected cultures of human fetal diploid cells. Proc. Soc. exp. Biol. (N. Y.) 116, 144—149 (1964).

SCHMIDT, N. J., E. H. LENNETTE, J. D. WOODIE, and H. H. HO: Immunofluorescent staining in the laboratory diagnosis of varicella-zoster virus infections. J. Lab. clin. Med. 66, 403—412 (1965 b).

SEIDENBERG, S.: Untersuchungen über das Herpes- und Zostervirus. Z. Hyg., Infekt.-Kr. 112, 134—150 (1931).

SEILER, H. E.: A study of herpes zoster particularly in its relationship to chickenpox. J. Hyg. (Lond.) 47, 253—262 (1949).

SELIGMAN, B. R., and F. ROSNER: Varicella and cytosine arabinoside. Lancet 1, 307—308 (1970).

SHANBROM, E., S. MILLER, and H. HAAR: Herpes zoster in hematologic neoplasias: some unusual manifestations. Ann. intern. Med. 53, 523—533 (1960).

SHAW, D. G.: Laboratory studies on varicella-zoster virus. Ph.D. Thesis, Liverpool University (1968).

SHAW, E. B., and M. GROSSMAN: Viral contagious infections. In: Pediatric Therapy, 2nd Edit. (H. C. SHIRKEY ed.), St. Louis: Mosby. Ch. 55, p. 410 (1966).

SIEGEL, M., and H. T. FUERST: Low birth weight and maternal virus diseases. A prospective study of rubella, measles, mumps, chickenpox and hepatitis. J. Amer. med. Ass. 197, 680—684 (1966).

SIEGEL, M., H. T. FUERST, and N. S. PERESS: Comparative fetal mortality in maternal virus diseases: a prospective study on rubella, measles, mumps, chickenpox and hepatitis. New Engl. J. Med. 274, 768—771 (1966).

SIMONS, J. S., T. F. WHAYNE, G. W. ANDERSON, and H. M. HORACK: Global Epidemiology. Philadelphia: J. B. Lippincott Co., 1944.

SIMPSON, R. E. H.: Infectiousness of communicable diseases in the household (measles, chickenpox and mumps). Lancet 2, 549—554 (1952).

SIMPSON, R. E. H.: Studies on shingles. Is the virus ordinary chickenpox virus? Lancet 2, 1299—1302 (1954).

SLOTNICK, V. B., and E. I. ROSANOFF: Localization of varicella virus in tissue culture. Virology 19, 589—592 (1963).

SMITH, I. W., J. F. PEUTHERER, and F. O. MacCALLUM: The incidence of herpesvirus hominis antibody in the population. J. Hyg. (Lond.) 65, 395—408 (1967).

SOKAL, J. E., and D. FIRAT: Varicella-zoster infection in Hodgkin's disease: clinical and epidemiological aspects. Amer. J. Med. 39, 452—463 (1965).

Söltz-Szöts, J.: Virologische und serologische Untersuchungen beim Herpes zoster. Arch. klin. exp. Derm. **220**, 105—128 (1964).

Söltz-Szöts, J.: Untersuchungen mit Varizellen-Herpes-zoster-Virus. Arch. klin. exp. Derm. **221**, 456—462 (1965).

Steiner: Zur Inokulation der Varizellen. Wien. med. Wschr. **25**, 306—308 (1875).

Stern, E. S.: The mechanism of herpes zoster and its relation to chicken-pox. Brit. J. Derm. **49**, 263—271 (1937).

Stevens, D. A., and T. C. Merigan: personal communication (1971).

Stokes, J.: "Varicella-Herpes Zoster group" In: Viral and Rickettsial Infections of Man 3rd Edition Ch. 39, 113—119 (T. M. Rivers and F. L. Horsfall, eds.). Philadelphia: Lippincott, 1959.

Ström, J.: Social development and declining incidence of some common epidemic diseases in children. A study of the incidence in different age groups in Stockholm. Acta paediat. (Uppsala) **56**, 159—163 (1967).

Suzuki, Y., M. Suzuki, and Y. Fukuyama: Neurological complications of varicella. Advanc. neurol. Sci. (Tokyo) **11**, 887—896 (1967).

Svedmyr, A.: Varicella virus in HeLa cells. Arch. ges. Virusforsch. **17**, 495—503 (1965).

Svedmyr, A.: Production of varicella-zoster CF antigen in a continuous line of Grivet kidney cells. Acta. path. microbiol. scand. **67**, 159—160 (1966).

Swan, C., and A. L. Tostevin: Congenital abnormalities in infants following infectious diseases during pregnancy, with special reference to rubella: a third series of cases. Med. J. Aust. **1**, 645—659 (1946).

Swan, C., A. L. Tostevin, and G. H. B. Black: Final observations on congenital defects in infants following infectious diseases during pregnancy, with special reference to rubella. Med. J. Aust. **2**, 889—908 (1946).

Taniguchi, T., M. Hosokawa, S. Kuga, and Z. Masuda: The virus of herpes and zoster. Jap. J. exp. Med. **12**, 101—104 (1934).

Taniguchi, T., Y. Kogita, M. Hosokawa, and S. Kuga: A cultivation of the vaccinia and varicella viruses in the chorio-allantoic membrane of the chick embryo, with special references to the preparation of the bacteria-free vaccine and prophylactic inoculation against varicella. Jap. J. exp. Med. **13**, 19—30 (1935).

Tausch, M.: Beitrag zum Vorkommen eines mit auf die Welt gebrachten Herpes zoster am Neugeborenen. Zbl. Gynäk. **56**, 1629—1633 (1932).

Tawara, J., and H. Ogiwara: Electron microscopic observations of the cells infected with Varicella-zoster virus. Jap. J. Microbiol. **13**, 37—50 (1969).

Taylor-Robinson, D.: Chickenpox and herpes zoster. MD Thesis. Liverpool University (1958).

Taylor-Robinson, D.: Chickenpox and herpes zoster. III. Tissue culture studies. Brit. J. exp. Path. **40**, 521—532 (1959).

Taylor-Robinson, D.: Herpes zoster occurring in a patient with chickenpox. Brit. med. J. **1**, 1713 (1960).

Taylor-Robinson, D., and A. W. Downie: Chickenpox and herpes zoster. I. Complement fixation studies. Brit. J. exp. Path. **40**, 398—409 (1959).

Taylor-Robinson, D., and C. J. M. Rondle: Chickenpox and herpes zoster. II. Ouchterlony precipitation studies. Brit. J. exp. Path. **40**, 517—520 (1959).

Taylor-Robinson, D., and D. A. J. Tyrrell: Virus diseases on Tristan da Cunha. Trans. roy. Soc. trop. Med. Hyg. **57**, 19—22 (1963).

Teague, O., and E. W. Goodpasture: Experimental herpes zoster. Preliminary report. J. Amer. med. Ass. **81**, 377—378 (1923).

Teixeria, de Castro-, J.: Infection de l'allanto-chorion de l'embryon de poulet par le virus de la varicelle. C. R. Soc. Biol. (Paris) **121**, 779—780 (1936 a).

Teixeria, de Castro-, J.: Infection de l'allanto-chorion de l'embryon de poulet par le virus de l'herpès zoster. C. R. Soc. Biol. (Paris) **121**, 781—782 (1936 b).

Thompson, B. E.: Variola or varicella? Med. J. Aust. **2**, 615—617 (1967).

Thomson, F. H.: The aerial conveyance of infection, with a note on the contact infection of chicken-pox. Lancet **1**, 341—344 (1916).

THOMSEN, O.: Komplementbindungsuntersuchungen bei Zoster und Varizellen. Z. Immunforsch. **82**, 88—94 (1934).

TOMLINSON, A. H., and F. O. MacCALLUM: The incidence of complement-fixing antibody to varicella-zoster virus in hospital patients and blood donors. J. Hyg. (Lond.) **68**, 411—416 (1970).

TOP, F. H.: Handbook of Communicable Diseases. St. Louis: C. V. Mosby, 1941.

TOURNIER, P., F. CATHALA, and W. BERNHARD: Ultrastructure et développement intracellulaire du virus de la varicelle observé au microscope électronique. Presse méd. **65**, 1229—1234 (1957).

TRIEBWASSER, J. H., R. E. HARRIS, R. E. BRYANT, and E. R. RHOADES: Varicella pneumonia in adults. Report of seven cases and a review of literature. Medicine (Baltimore) **46**, 409—423 (1967).

TRIMBLE, G. X.: Attenuation of chickenpox with gamma globulin. Canad. med. Ass. J. **77**, 697—699 (1957).

TRLIFAJOVÁ, J., J. ŠOUREK, and M. RYBA: Preparation of concentrated intracellular precipitating antigens of varicella-zoster and herpes simplex viruses and results obtained with them in the gel precipitation reaction. Acta virol. **14**, 25—34 (1970).

TYZZER, E. E.: The histology of the skin lesions in varicella. J. med. Res. **14**, 361—392 (1905—1906).

TZANCK, A., and R. ARON-BRUNETIÈRE: Le cyto diagnostic immédiat des dermatoses bulleuses. Gaz. méd. port. **2**, 667—675 (1949).

UNDERWOOD, E. A.: The neurologic complications of varicella: a clinical and epidemiological study. Brit. J. Child. Dis. **32**, 83—107; 177—196; 241—263 (1935).

UNNA, P. G.: The Histopathology of the Diseases of the Skin. Edinburgh: W. F. Clay, 149—154 (1896).

VÁCZI, L., L. GÉDER, M. KOLLER, and E. JENEY: Influence of temperature on the multiplication of varicella virus. Acta microbiol. hung. **10**, 109—115 (1963).

VALLONE, E. F., R. M. CANTO, and R. E. SOMMA: Varicella and corticoids. Virologic and clinical aspects. Arch. Pediat. Urug. **36**, 296—306 (1965 a).

VALLONE, E. F., R. M. CANTO, and R. E. SOMMA: Isolation of varicella virus on chick embryo chorioallantoic membrane. An. Fac. Med. Montevideo **50**, 169—175 (1965 b).

VAN ROOYEN, C. E., and R. S. ILLINGWORTH: A laboratory test for the diagnosis of smallpox. Brit. med. J., **2**, 526—529 (1944).

VAN ROOYEN, C. E., and A. J. RHODES: Virus Diseases of Man. 2nd Ed. New York: Thomas Nelson and Sons, 1948.

VASILENKO, P. V.: On the causative agent of herpes zoster. Vestn. Derm. Vener. **40**, 16—20 (1966).

WALTUCH, G., and F. SACHS: Herpes zoster in a patient with Hodgkin's disease: treatment with iododeoxyuridine. Arch. intern. Med. **121**, 458—462 (1968).

WARING, J. J., K. NEUBUERGER, and E. F. GEEVER: Severe forms of chickenpox in adults with autopsy observations in a case with associated pneumonia and encephalitis. Arch. intern. Med. **69**, 384—408 (1942).

WEECH, A. A.: The prophylaxis of varicella with convalescents' serum. J. Amer. med. Ass. **82**, 1245—1246 (1924).

WEINGARTEN, C. M.: A renewed plea for the isolation of shingles. Report of a case. Dis. Chest **47**, 451 (1965).

WEINTRAUB, I. I.: Treatment of herpes zoster with gamma globulin. J. Amer. med. Ass. **157**, 1611 (1955).

WELLER, T. H.: Serial propagation *in vitro* of agents producing inclusion bodies derived from varicella and herpes zoster. Proc. Soc. exp. Biol. (N. Y.) **83**, 340—346 (1953).

WELLER, T. H.: Discussion in Proceedings of the decennial review conference on tissue culture. J. nat. Cancer Inst. **19**, 702—704 (1957).

WELLER, T. H.: Observations on the behaviour of certain viruses that produce intranuclear inclusion bodies in man. The Harvey Lectures. Series 52, pp. 228—254, 1956—1957 (1958).

WELLER, T. H.: "Varicella-herpes zoster virus" In: Viral and Rickettsial Infections of Man. 4th Edition Ch. 42, 915—925 (F. L. HORSFALL and I. TAMM eds.). Philadelphia: Lippincott, 1965.

WELLER, T. H.: Prospects for immunization against varicella and cytomegalovirus infections. 1st Int. Conf. on Vaccines against Viral and Rickettsial Infections of Man. pp. 276—282 (1967).

WELLER, T. H.: Varicella-zoster virus. In: Diagnostic Procedures for Viral and Rickettsial Infections. 4th Edition Ch. 21, pp. 733—754 (E. H. LENNETTE and N. J. SCHMIDT eds.) Amer. Publ. Hlth Ass., N. Y. (1969).

WELLER, T. H., and A. H. COONS: Fluorescent antibody studies with agents of varicella and herpes zoster propagated in vitro. Proc. Soc. exp. Biol. (N. Y.) 86, 789—794 (1954).

WELLER, T. H., and M. B. STODDARD: Intranuclear inclusion bodies in cultures of human tissue inoculated with varicella vesicle fluid. J. Immunol. 68, 311—319 (1952).

WELLER, T. H., and H. M. WITTON: The etiologic agents of varicella and herpes zoster. Serologic studies with the viruses as propagated in vitro. J. exp. Med. 108, 869—890 (1958).

WELLER, T. H., H. M. WITTON, and E. J. BELL: The etiologic agents of varicella and herpes zoster. Isolation, propagation, and cultural characteristics in vitro. J. exp. Med. 108, 843—868 (1958).

WELLS, W. F., M. W. WELLS, and T. S. WILDER: The environmental control of epidemic contagion. I. An epidemiologic study of radiant disinfection of air in day schools. Amer. J. Hyg. 35, 97—121 (1942).

WENNER, H. A., and T. Y. LOU: Virus diseases associated with cutaneous eruptions Progr. med. Virol. 5, 219—294 (1963).

WESSELHOEFT, C.: The differential diagnosis of chickenpox and smallpox. New Engl. J. Med. 230, 15—19 (1944).

WESSELHOEFT, C., and C. M. PEARSON: Orchitis in the course of severe chickenpox with pneumonitis, followed by testicular atrophy. New Engl. J. Med. 242, 651—656 (1950).

WHEELOCK, E. F.: The role of interferon in human viral infections. 1st Int. Conf. on Vaccines against Viral and Rickettsial Infections of Man. pp. 623—631 (1967).

WILE, U. J., and H. H. HOLMAN: Generalized herpes zoster associated with leukemia. Arch. Derm. Syph. (Chic.) 42, 587—592 (1940).

WILKINSON, J. S.: Abitylguanide (ABOB) in treating herpes zoster. N. C. med. J. 23, 357—360 (1962).

WILLÉN, R., R. BERG, O. HANSSON, F. NORDBRING, P. SOURANDER, and U. STENRAM: Fatal varicella generalisata in a child with immunopathy and neurological retardation. Acta path. microbiol. scand. 72, 448—449 (1968).

WILLIAMS, B., and T. H. CAPERS: The demonstration of intranuclear inclusion bodies in sputum from a patient with varicella pneumonia. Amer. J. Med. 27, 836—839 (1959).

WILLIAMS, M. G., J. D. ALMEIDA, and A. F. HOWATSON: Electron microscope studies on viral skin lesions. A simple and rapid method of identifying virus particles. Arch. Derm. Syph. (Chic.) 86, 290—297 (1962).

WINKELMANN, R. K., and H. O. PERRY: Herpes zoster in children. J. Amer. med. Ass. 171, 376—380 (1959).

WOHLWILL, F.: Zur pathologischen Anatomie des Nervensystems beim Herpes Zoster (auf Grund von zehn Sektionsfällen). Z. ges. Neurol. Psychiat. 89, 171—212 (1924).

WOOLLEY, E. J. S.: Herpes zoster in an isolated community. Brit. med. J. 1, 392 (1946).

WRIGHT, E. T., and L. H. WINER: Herpes zoster and malignancy. Arch. Derm. 84, 242—244 (1961).

YAMADA, K., Y. YOKOTA, H. KAWAI, and Y. AOYAMA: Varicella pneumonia with hypogamma-globulinaemia. Med. J. Shinshu Univ. 13, 9—21 (1968).

YUCEOGLU, A. M., S. BERKOVICH, and S. MINKOWITZ: Acute glomerulonephritis as a complication of varicella. J. Amer. med. Ass. 202, 879—881 (1967).

VIROLOGY MONOGRAPHS

DIE VIRUSFORSCHUNG IN EINZELDARSTELLUNGEN

VIROLOGY
MONOGRAPHS
DIE VIRUSFORSCHUNG IN EINZELDARSTELLUNGEN

Further volumes in preparation. / Weitere Bände in Vorbereitung.